Thyroid Problems

THYROID PROBLEMS

A guide to symptoms and treatments

Patsy Westcott

Thorsons
An Imprint of HarperCollins*Publishers*

Thorsons
An Imprint of HarperCollins*Publishers*
77–85 Fulham Palace Road,
Hammersmith, London W6 8JB
1160 Battery Street,
San Francisco, California 94111–1213

Published by Thorsons 1995
1 3 5 7 9 10 8 6 4 2

A catalogue record for this book
is available from the British Library

ISBN 0 7225 3164 8

Printed in Great Britain by
HarperCollinsManufacturing Glasgow

CONTENTS

ACKNOWLEDGEMENTS

Many people have helped with this book. The biggest and most heartfelt thank-you goes to the hundreds of women who replied to my advert in *The Guardian* and who shared their experience of thyroid disease so honestly – without whom nothing.

I should like to thank Claire Lower of the British Medical Association for her help with research. Thanks, too, to Janis Hickey of the British Thyroid Foundation for discussing thyroid problems and supplying me with leaflets and newsletters. Professor Lazarus and Professor Weetman also helped by telling me about their research and sharing their thoughts on thyroid disease.

Finally, thank you to my daughter, Lucy Westcott, who supplied the illustrations at such short notice.

Chapter 1

THE HIDDEN ILLNESS

Why a book on thyroid problems for women? Well, read the following sentence:

> *Thyroid disease is common and affects women more frequently than men.*

Many chapters on thyroid disease in books written for both lay readers and the medical profession begin with some such observation, yet this bland statement barely begins to hint at the numbers of women afflicted by thyroid disease or the impact it can have on their lives.

In terms of statistics alone, thyroid problems deserve to be taken more seriously. Consider the following facts:

- According to UK endocrinologist Dr Paul Belchetz, writing in the newsletter of the British Thyroid Foundation, 'Perhaps one in ten women at some stage in their life will suffer from some form of thyroid disorder'.
- It's been estimated that perhaps as many as a million people in the UK suffer from autoimmune thyroid disease alone,

which is when the body turns against itself, causing the thyroid to become either under- or overactive.

- Five women to every man suffer from Hashimoto's thyroiditis – one such autoimmune thyroid disorder – which causes the thyroid to become underactive.
- Graves' disease, which causes the thyroid to become overactive, is 15 times more likely to affect women than men.
- Thyroid disease can affect women at any age or stage in life, from the teen years to retirement age, but is most common during the reproductive years.
- One in ten young women have thyroid problems after giving birth to a baby, suffering depression, tiredness and a general lack of zest, which can mar the first months of parenthood. Such problems are often misdiagnosed as 'the baby blues', depriving women of treatment that would help them.
- In later life, thyroid disease is associated with an increased risk of two very significant causes of ill-health in women: heart disease and the brittle bone disease, osteoporosis, both of which strike after the menopause. Both deprive women of the chance to actively enjoy their later years and, tragically, are also the cause of much illness and death in later life.

The figures alone put thyroid disease on a par with such high-profile illnesses as diabetes (estimated to affect 1 to 2 in every 100) and breast cancer, which strikes 1 in 12. These attract huge amounts of research funds and many column inches in magazines and newspapers, yet thyroid problems remain largely ignored. Granted, thyroid disease isn't life-threatening, but it is still the cause of much depression, tiredness, discomfort and feelings of being under par, especially as women often soldier on for months and sometimes years before anyone takes their complaints seriously. In the UK, at the time of writing, there are just three books for lay people on thyroid disease, compared with shelves full on problems with a similar incidence, and none of them is aimed solely at women.

I have to admit that, despite many years of writing about women's health, until I came to research this book, I had no idea just how common thyroid problems are or of the misery they can cause. However, when I put a small notice in *The Guardian*, requesting women who had suffered thyroid problems to contact me, I was deluged: 200 phone calls within 2 days. All too many of these women had struggled on for months, sometimes years, with crippling symptoms before being diagnosed. Once diagnosed, they had to face treatments that were uncertain in action, took time to get right or sometimes didn't work at all.

Some related the dilemmas posed by treatment – how long it had taken for treatment to start working, the difficulties of deciding whether or not to opt for surgery. Others agonized about the effects of radioactive iodine, a treatment for an overactive thyroid. They told of the difficulties of getting information relevant to their needs and of how alone they felt with this unpredictable disease.

Others I spoke to told poignant stories of how the disease had affected their daily lives, of how it felt to be overweight because of an underactive thyroid, of the self-consciousness they endured because of bulging eyes, thinning hair and thickened skin, and of the effects these changes had on their self-esteem. Some described the heartache of not being recognized by friends they hadn't seen for a while.

Such physical problems are often dismissed as being trivial. However, in a world where women are so often judged on their looks, they can be the cause of much misery. They can also lead on to other female health problems such as eating disorders. For example, a recent study of female thyroid disease sufferers, for example, revealed that they are at a far higher risk of developing anorexia and bulimia than other women. Twice as many women suffering from thyroid problems (1 in 25 female thyroid sufferers) are bulimic, locked into a helpless cycle of bingeing and dieting.

The researchers suggest that weight swings brought about by thyroid disease and treatment, together with distressing changes in physical appearance, add up to a negative body image, so that sufferers become obsessed with the scales, feeling that their weight is the only factor they can control.

The Tip of the Iceberg?

In recent years, doctors have begun to suspect that thyroid problems could be even more common than was ever imagined. The advent of more sophisticated biochemical tests has revealed that as many as 15 per cent of seemingly perfectly healthy older women and 2 per cent of other individuals with apparently normal thyroid function have antibodies against thyroid tissue in their blood. This suggests that the thyroid disease that is picked up and treated is only a fraction of that which actually exists.

Such 'silent' or subclinical thyroid disease – the terms used to describe problems that don't cause any obvious symptoms – is the subject of intense debate among experts, especially in the USA. Around 1 in 10 women aged over 40 are diagnosed as having it. This is important because the disease is known to raise cholesterol levels in the blood – one of the major risk factors for heart disease. Given that women are more prone to developing heart problems as they get older, which are often not picked up and treated, could this be something to do with undiagnosed thyroid malfunction? And how important is such hidden thyroid disease as a cause of depression and fatigue or debilitating problems such as weight gain, dry skin and hair, and constipation? How often does it lead to overt thyroid disease? Should it be screened for? And should it be treated? Such questions have still not been answered.

Why Me?

Almost every woman I spoke to wanted to know *why* they had developed thyroid disease. Unfortunately, there are no simple answers. Despite its prevalence, the experts themselves still don't fully understand what causes the thyroid to misbehave. As with so many illnesses one of the most pressing questions is, is nature or nurture to blame? Genes undoubtedly play a part, but so too does the environment. Many aspects of twentieth-century life seem to have a role in the development of thyroid disease. The immune system, ageing, diet, stress and virus or bacterial infections are just some of the factors currently being explored by researchers in the hope of finding out why the thyroid becomes faulty.

The Immune Connection

The role played by the immune system in sparking off a number of thyroid disorders is one of the hottest topics of research. Autoimmune thyroid disease, which, as already observed, lies behind swings to both over- and underactivity, is caused by a failure of one of the body's most basic mechanisms: recognizing its own organs and tissues as belonging to itself. It's this process, known as immunity, that protects us against disease. If the body *fails* to recognize itself, it attacks its own tissue, causing an autoimmune disease. The experts are increasingly realizing that a number of very diverse thyroid problems are caused by the body producing antibodies against the thyroid tissue. These include:

- Hashimoto's disease – underactivity of the thyroid gland
- myxoedema – tissue swelling, caused by underactivity of the thyroid

- silent thyroiditis – inflammation of the thyroid gland, caused by overactivity, which is not accompanied by any pain or discomfort in the thyroid
- subclinical hypothyroidism – underactivity of the thyroid without any overt symptoms, which, in some cases, leads on to overt hypothyroidism
- post-partum thyroiditis – inflammation of the thyroid coming on after childbirth
- Graves' disease – overactivity of the thyroid gland

A Genetic Link?

Women tend to be the guardians of their family's health, as wives, mothers, sisters and daughters, and thyroid problems often run in families. Women are also, as we've seen, the major sufferers of thyroid disease. Many of the sufferers I spoke to said, almost as an afterthought, 'My mother suffers from thyroid problems, too'. In particular, Graves' disease and Hashimoto's disease – respectively over- and underactivity of thyroid – seem to cluster in families. In the past, this was dismissed as coincidence. In recent years, however, the interest in the part played by autoimmunity has led a number of scientists to search for an underlying genetic factor. The result, it's now being suggested, is that possession of antibodies against thyroid tissue is a trait, just like blue eyes, that is determined by a gene dominant in women.

But genes aren't the whole story as many people possess such antibodies *without* developing full-blown thyroid disease. As with so many genetically linked problems, the genes load the gun, but the environment pulls the trigger. The experts are thus also trying to find out what the possible triggers could be. We know that the immune system can be damaged by many aspects of modern life – increased pollution, viruses and other infections, smoking, drinking and, above all, stress. Scientists are investigating all these factors as triggers in thyroid disease, but one factor could simply lie in the fact of being female.

The Hormonal Connection

The thyroid is involved in practically every bodily process, including those of the reproductive system. Thyroid disease frequently strikes between the ages of 20 and 40 – the fertile years – and is often linked to a number of specifically female problems, as shown below.

A Women's Problem?

Symptoms of hypothyroidism (underactivity of the thyroid)	*Symptoms of hyperthyroidism (overactivity of the thyroid)*
Menstruation	**Menstruation**
• PMS (further research is required to confirm this) • Loss of periods • Heavy periods in mild cases	• Irregular periods, scanty flow • Loss of periods in severe cases
Fertility	**Fertility**
• Lack of ovulation • Recurrent miscarriage	• No major effect in mild to moderate cases • Recurrent miscarriage in severe cases

The first clue that something may be wrong with the thyroid is often when a women visits the doctor for some 'women's problem'. For example, because of period irregularities, difficulty in getting pregnant, during pregnancy or after having a baby. It's even been suggested that mild overactivity of the thyroid gland could play a part in PMS (premenstrual syndrome).

Many of the conditions produce a goitre (a swollen or enlarged thyroid gland), which is four times as common among women as men. It's common and quite normal for the thyroid to enlarge slightly during the teens and early adult life and also during pregnancy, causing the neck to appear slightly bigger than usual. Some women notice a slight tightness around the neckline of close-fitting blouses or sweaters just before their period starts, too – a sign that the thyroid is mildly enlarged. And a slight enlargement of the thyroid is also fairly common around the menopause. It's quite possible to have a goitre that causes no problems whatsoever – a simple non-toxic goitre – but sometimes a goitre is linked to abnormal secretion of hormones, caused by either under- or overactivity.

With so many women's problems being linked to thyroid disease and, conversely, so many thyroid problems being associated with the reproductive cycle, could it be that female hormones themselves have a part to play in increasing women's susceptibility to thyroid disease? The answer seems to be yes. The sex hormones, of which oestrogen is one of the main female ones, are recognized to have an effect on the immune system. Studies in animals show that oestrogens make inflammation of the thyroid (thyroiditis) worse, while testosterone, the male sex hormone, improves it.

Other research has shown that another female hormone, prolactin, also plays a role in the development of thyroid disease. Changed levels of these hormones and the other changes in the immune system that occur during pregnancy could account for the fact that autoimmune thyroid problems tend to ease off during the final months of pregnancy, only to flare up with renewed vigour after birth. The involvement of hormones could also explain why normally symptomless thyroid problems often become apparent for the first time after birth. It also suggests a reason for so many women developing inflammation of the gland, together with symptoms of over- and/or underactivity, a condition called post-partum thyroiditis (PPT), after giving birth. Researchers are looking at the links between the development of PPT and postnatal depression, estimated to strike as many as one in ten women after having a baby.

With Women in Mind

This book – the first to deal specifically with thyroid problems in women – explores these and other issues. As a medical journalist, I believe that the more you know about the way your body works, the better you are able to help yourself if something goes wrong. In this book, I aim to give you the information you need to enable you to help yourself, to work with your doctor so that you can get the best treatment for your situation, and to give you back a feeling of control over your body and your life (something women with thyroid problems often feel they have lost).

The next chapter kicks off by looking in some detail at the thyroid gland itself and how it works. Reading it should enable you to understand just why when the thyroid goes wrong it can have such wide-ranging effects.

Chapters 3 and 4 look at underactivity and overactivity of the thyroid gland and explore some of the latest theories about how they arise in an attempt to answer that nagging question, 'Why me?'

Chapter 5 is devoted to thyroid eye disease, a particularly distressing condition.

This is followed in Chapter 6 by a thorough run-down of how

thyroid disease affects pregnancy and childbirth, and looks at post-partum thyroiditis, which strikes as many as 15 per cent of women after birth.

Chapter 7 tackles the difficulties of getting a diagnosis.

This is followed in Chapter 8 by a run-down of the various types of treatment, explaining how they work, the pros and cons and how you can decide what is right for you.

One of the worst aspects of having a chronic illness is the lack of control sufferers often feel, so Chapters 9 and 10 cover the different ways in which women can get a grip on the situation. The first of these looks at some simple ways in which you can help yourself, and how to come to terms psychologically with having thyroid disease. The second includes details of the ways in which alternative and complementary therapies might be able to help.

The final chapter, Chapter 11, looks at some of the current pressing issues in thyroid disease, at new advances in our understanding of it, and attempts to take a peek into the future at the possible new treatments.

Chapter 2

How the Thyroid Works

The thyroid is a small, soft gland, weighing just 15 to 20 g (½ to ¾ oz). It is one of ten glands that make up the endocrine, or hormonal, system. From the moment we are conceived until we die, our bodies are under the influence of a cocktail of hormones produced by these glands. This system is so finely tuned that when anything happens to disturb its delicate balance, the repercussions ricochet throughout the rest of the body.

The hormones produced by the glands are chemical messengers, which are carried around the bloodstream to act on cells and tissues that are often far from their site of origin. Their job is to ensure that we have the right concentration of metabolites – vital nutrients (sugars, fatty acids, vitamins and minerals, such as calcium, sodium, potassium and iodine, enzymes) and other factors essential to life – in our bloodstream.

Each gland has its own specific function, also working with other glands in the body. As we develop from baby to child to adult, for instance, our growth is regulated by a hormone called somatotrophin that is produced by the pituitary gland, by the thyroid hormones thyroxine and triiodothyronine, and by hormones produced by the reproductive glands, controlled by the pituitary.

Key Sites

The glands themselves are situated in key areas throughout our bodies. The pituitary is in the head, the thyroid and parathyroids in the neck, the thymus at the top of the chest, the adrenals and the pancreas in the abdomen, and the gonads, or reproductive glands, in the pelvis (see Figure 2.1).

Together they produce over 50 different hormones, and, as these cannot be stored in large quantities in the glands themselves, the brain programmes the glands to manufacture the hormones by means of a complicated biochemical cycle, designed to keep the body in a state of balance or homeostasis.

Not surprisingly, with such a complicated gland, quite a few things can go wrong. However, whatever the underlying causes, broadly speaking, problems fall into two categories. The gland may become underactive and produce too few hormones, a condition described as hypothyroidism ('hypo' meaning 'below' or 'too little'). Alternatively, the thyroid can become overactive and produce too many hormones. In this case, the term used is hyperthyroidism ('hyper' meaning 'above' or 'too much'). Hyperthyroidism is also known as thyrotoxicosis (literally, thyroid poisoning). Although hypothyroidism and hyperthyroidism sound similar, the two conditions couldn't be more different. What they share, however, is that they affect so many of the body's systems.

Balancing the Body

The whole homeostasis process is controlled by a series of 'feedback loops' that slow or stop the gland from working once enough of a hormone has been produced and turn it on again when more is needed, rather like the way in which a central heating thermostat operates (see Figure 2.2). When a room reaches

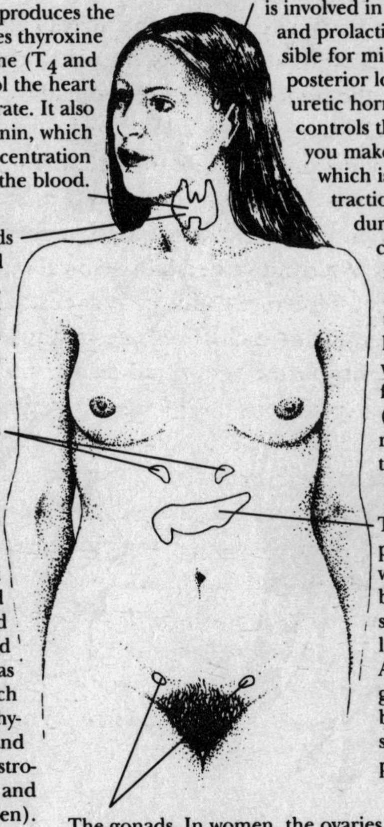

The pituitary gland – just the size of a peanut – controls the actions of all the other glands in the body. Its anterior lobe produces growth hormone, which is involved in growth and ageing, and prolactin, which is responsible for milk production. Its posterior lobe produces antidiuretic hormone (ADH), which controls the amount of urine you make, and oxytocin, which is involved in contractions of the uterus during pregnancy, childbirth and breastfeeding. The pituitary also produces thyroid stimulating hormone (TSH), which triggers the flow of thyroxine (T_4) and triiodothyronine (T_3) from the thyroid.

The thyroid gland produces the thyroid hormones thyroxine and triiodothyronine (T_4 and T_3), which control the heart and metabolic rate. It also produces calcitonin, which regulates the concentration of calcium in the blood.

The parathyroid glands produce parathyroid hormone (PTH), which regulates the turnover of calcium and phosphorus in the bones.

The adrenal glands consist of two organs. The first produces the stress hormones adrenaline and noradrenaline, which regulate heart rate and blood pressure. The second produce steroid hormones, such as hydrocortisone, which help convert carbohydrate into energy, and the sex hormones oestrogen, progesteron and testosterone (in men). These control sexual development, fertility and reproduction.

The pancreas produces insulin, which helps maintain blood sugar levels. A shortage of insulin leads to diabetes. Another hormone, glucagon, produced by the pancreas, stimulates the liver to produce glucose.

The gonads. In women, the ovaries produce the sex hormones oestrogen and progesterone, which control the menstrual cycle and reproduction. (In men, the equivalent is the prostate gland, which produces the male sex hormone, testosterone).

***Figure 2.1** The endocrine system*

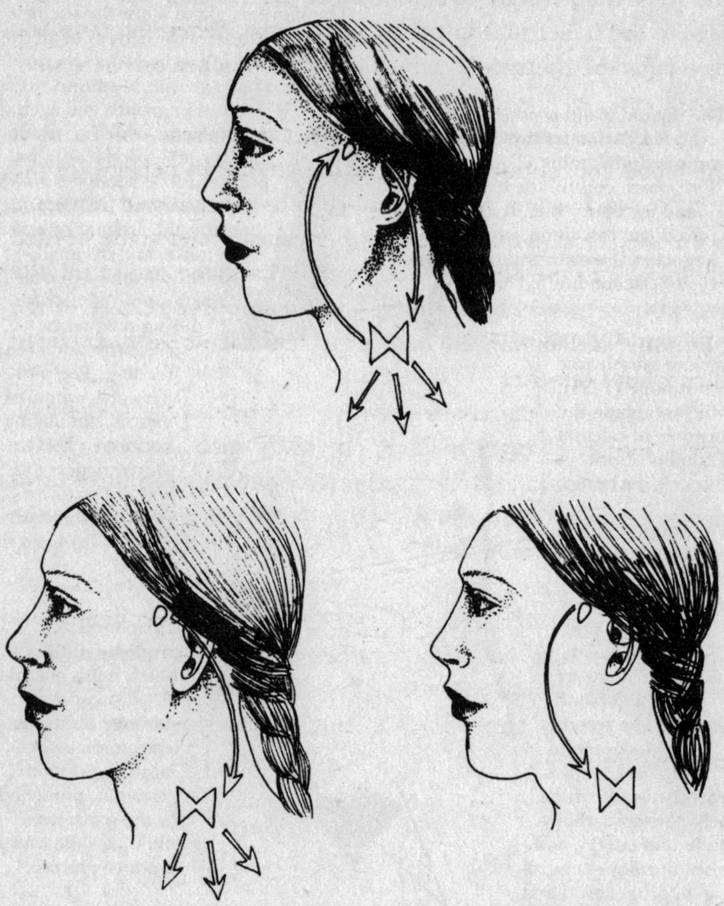

Figure 2.2 The pituitary gland and the hypothalamus in the brain work together to produce a hormone that stimulates the thyroid. The thyroid gland draws iodine from the blood in order to make T_3 and T_4. Sensors in the TSH-secreting cells of the pituitary detect rising levels of thyroid hormones and quell further secretion. When levels fall, the pituitary releases more TSH, which stimulates the thyroid to start making more hormones.

the right temperature, a sensor in the thermostat relays a message to the boiler to stop pumping out heat. When the temperature falls, the thermostat senses this and switches on the system again.

In a similar way, sensory cells in the body possess a set point. If the blood concentration of any of the chemicals needed for the body to work is low, these receptive cells sense it and release a hormone. This, in turn, acts on other cells to release the needed chemical into the blood. When enough has been produced, the receptive cells switch off the system, so stopping release of the hormone. In this way, the body's internal balance is maintained throughout our lives.

The system is extremely sensitive: the food we eat, exercise, stress, illness, changes in body chemistry such as shortages or excesses of certain nutrients, pregnancy, ageing, even the time of day or year, can affect the balancing mechanism and with it the amounts of hormones the glands secrete.

Most hormones are responsible for acting only on specific tissues, not all the cells in the body. They do this by latching on to special 'receptors', which are on the surface of or inside cells, in a similar way to how a key fits into a lock, and this enables the hormones to be transported around the bloodstream to their destination.

The Thyroid Gland

The thyroid itself is a butterfly-shaped gland situated across the front of the windpipe, or trachea, just below the larynx, or voice box (see Figure 2.3). It consists of two lobes or sections that lie on either side of the Adam's apple, joined together by a bridge of glandular tissue called the isthmus.

If you are young and slim, you may just be able to detect the outline of your thyroid if you look in the mirror and stretch your

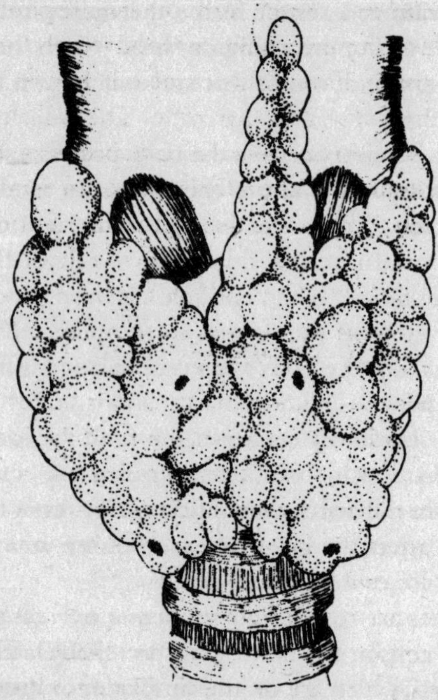

Figure 2.3 The thyroid gland lies across the windpipe in the throat.

neck. If you then swallow, you may be able to see it moving up and down. If you can't see it, you may be able to feel it if you probe your neck with your fingers. (Don't worry if you can't see *or* feel it though – only about half of us can.)

The gland develops in the first weeks of life from a small piece of tissue at the root of the tongue. As the unborn baby grows, this piece of tissue moves down the neck via a narrow passage called the thyroglossal duct to its adult position. By the time the fetus is just 12 weeks old, the thyroid gland has already started to work.

The tissue that makes up the thyroid gland is made up of two types of hormone-secreting cells: follicular cells and parafollicular cells. The follicular cells, which form the largest part, are hollow spheres, surrounded by tiny capillary blood vessels, lymph vessels and connective tissue. These follicles secrete the two thyroid hormones, triiodothyronine and thyroxine. The follicles are filled with a yellow, semi-fluid, protein-containing material. The parafollicular cells are found on their own or in small clusters in the spaces between follicles and secrete another hormone, called calcitonin.

All Under Control

Like all the glands in the body, the thyroid is under the control of the pituitary gland, which lies at the base of the brain. This, in turn, is driven by a region of the brain called the hypothalamus, which is joined to the pituitary by a short stalk of nerve fibres. It's the job of the hypothalamus to coordinate the function of the nervous and endocrine systems in the body.

In the case of the thyroid, it does this by producing a chemical called thyrotropin releasing hormone (TRH). This triggers the pituitary into secreting thyroid stimulating hormone (TSH), and this, in turn, sparks the release of thyroxine (T_4) and triiodothyronine (T_3).

A Tale of Two Hormones

In fact, although there are two hormones, only T_3 is actually active on the cells. There is about 50 times more T_4 within the bloodstream than T_3. Once T_4 has travelled around the bloodstream to distant tissues, it is converted to T_3. For this reason, doctors and scientists tend to talk about thyroid hormone rather than thyroid hormones. The process of conversion is a bit like drawing on a deposit account at the bank for funds for your current account.

The Calcium Connection

As we saw, the parafollicular cells of the thyroid produce the hormone calcitonin, and it is involved in regulating calcium levels in the body. As well as being the main mineral used for the manufacture of bone, calcium is needed to trigger impulses in nerve and muscle cells and to maintain calcium levels in the blood.

Calcitonin acts with another hormone, parathyroid hormone (PTH), produced by the parathyroids, which are four tiny glands situated behind the thyroid gland. Whenever calcium is needed by the body, PTH raises blood levels of calcium by stimulating the release of calcium from the bone, increasing reabsorption of calcium from the kidneys and converting vitamin D into a hormone that increases gut absorption of calcium. Once calcium levels have been increased in this way, the thyroid releases calcitonin, which suppresses the release of any more of the mineral from the bone.

The Incredible Thyroid

Although the thyroid is small – around the size of a plum – the hormones produced by it are responsible for an amazing number of bodily processes. In fact, so widespread is the activity of the thyroid that, in Victorian times, doctors believed it was vital to life itself. It's now known that this was a false assumption: you can live without a thyroid, but only if you are given artificial replacements of thyroid hormone. Even so, thyroid hormones are unique in that, throughout our lives, they act within almost every tissue of the body.

A Matter of Energy

The main job of your thyroid is to control the metabolism (the speed of activity) of each of your body's cells. Thyroid hormones activate mitochondria, the tiny powerhouses of cells that produce energy. It's the process of metabolism – the word literally means 'change' – that, among other things, controls your appetite and ensures that your body remains at more or less the same temperature, whatever the outside environment.

Within the body, your metabolism determines the rate at which your cells burn up oxygen, a process involved in every single action of everyday life – from breathing, to eating, sleeping, talking and moving around, as well as all the activities of your internal organs, such as the beating of your heart, the process of digestion, the functioning of your reproductive organs and the working of your brain.

The Growth Factor

Thyroid hormones are vital for mental and physical growth. Together with somatotrophin (STH) from the pituitary, they determine the length and strength of your bones. During childhood, lack of thyroid hormones stunts growth by preventing the bones from growing and maturing. Thyroid hormones are also crucial for the normal development of your brain and nervous system. During pregnancy, thyroid hormones cross the placenta and low levels of one (T_4) can damage the development of the unborn baby's brain, causing cretinism (from which we get the word 'cretin', meaning 'mentally deficient').

Breast Development

Thyroid hormones may also be involved in the development of our breasts. (In mice they work with prolactin, another pituitary hormone, to regulate the development of the mammary gland.)

Transformation

Each of the millions of cells in our bodies becomes more specialized as it progresses to maturity. In so doing, the cell develops the characteristics and functions unique to the tissue or organ to which it belongs – a process known as differentiation. It's this process that turns tadpoles into frogs, and, in human beings, causes the embryo to develop from a tiny cluster of cells to a fully grown baby.

At the beginning of life, the cells of the embryo are undifferentiated, but as the embryo begins to grow and develop, the cells begin to become more specialized. Thyroid hormones are believed to play a crucial part in controlling this process. In fact, without T_4 tadpoles don't develop into frogs.

Starvation Protection

When it works properly, the thyroid plays a crucial part in protecting us against starvation and keeping us at a more or less stable weight. Stepping up the amount you eat, especially of starchy foods or carbohydrates, increases the metabolism and boosts the production of the active thyroid hormone, T_3. Dieting, or cutting out starchy foods, on the other hand, decreases metabolism, causing the body to produce less T_3. This is almost certainly a protective mechanism, developed by our bodies to tide us over periods of starvation. It's a known fact that when human beings are deprived of food, the body turns down the metabolism. This is one of the mechanisms thought to have enabled the survival of the Mexican babies who were, incredibly, found to be still alive after several days of being trapped under rubble after the earthquake in Mexico City in the 1980s.

The Thyroid and Ageing

The thyroid is also believed to play a crucial part in controlling the process of growing older and, again, this is likely to be at least partly due to its effect on metabolism. In animals, limiting food intake has been found to slow down ageing and lower the incidence of age-linked degenerative illnesses. It's not known whether cutting calories has the same effect in humans, though US researchers are looking into just this question. Nor is it known quite what mechanism is involved, though it's thought that the immune system may be involved in some way. However, given their central role in the body and their links with metabolism and the immune system it is almost certain that thyroid hormones are part of the equation.

Protection Against Infection

The thyroid is also a vital part of the body's immune defence mechanism. It stimulates special cells found in the lymph nodes known as T cells, which help the body to fight against disease. An increasing amount of research is now focused on the role of the immune system in thyroid disease, as it's realized that many thyroid diseases are caused by autoimmunity, which, you will recall, is when the body fails to recognize its own tissues as belonging to itself and begins to produce antibodies against them, as you can see from the list of different types of goitre shown below.

Varieties of Goitre

If you have a goitre it may be one of the following kinds:

- simple non-toxic goitre – a simple swelling that doesn't affect thyroid function
- endemic goitre – the commonest cause worldwide, which results from lack of iodine
- autoimmune thyroid disease, such as Graves' disease – caused by overactivity – and Hashimoto's disease – caused by underactivity
- drug induced – caused by medically prescribed drugs, for example antithyroid drugs such as carbimazole, certain healthfood supplements such as kelp tablets, multivitamin and mineral preparations containing iodine, or amiodarone, prescribed for irregular heartbeat
- defects in enzymes involved in the synthesis of thyroid hormones, such as Pendred's syndrome
- thyroiditis – inflammation of the thyroid sometimes caused by

a virus (de Quervain's thyroiditis) or scarring and hardening of the thyroid tissue (Riedel's thyroiditis) as a result of autoimmunity
- thyroid adenoma – harmless swelling of a clump of cells or nodule
- carcinoma – cancerous swelling of thyroid cells, an extremely rare cause of goitre (5 to 10 per cent of single nodules) and usually easily curable.

Fluid Balance

As well as all the actions so far described, the thyroid plays a vital role in myriad other bodily processes. It is involved in fluid balance in the body by controlling the mechanisms by which fluids and chemicals enter and leave the cells.

Vitamin Power

In the liver, thyroid hormones are needed to convert beta-carotene (the pigment that gives orange, yellow and red fruits and vegetables their colour) into vitamin A. In the past few years, beta-carotene has stirred up a lot of interest as one of the three main antioxidant vitamins (the other two are vitamins C and E), which are thought to play a crucial role in protecting the body against degenerative diseases such as cancer and heart disease, and ageing.

Permissive Actions

Thyroid hormones are also needed to permit other hormones to act in various parts of the body. For example, in the brain, thyroid hormones allow the pituitary hormone, STH, to act. In pregnancy and throughout your reproductive life, they act with the female sex hormone, oestrogen. Thyroid malfunction is one relatively rare cause of female infertility, due to its effects on the reproductive hormones.

The Iodine Connection

The mineral iodine – a trace element found in the soil and present in the food we eat – plays a central role in the manufacture of thyroid hormones. Iodine is a metabolite, a chemical needed for cells to work. On average, our bodies contain around 20 to 30 milligrams, most of which is concentrated in the thyroid. To achieve this level, we need to take in about 100 to 200 micrograms a day from food (for sources of iodine, see below).

Know Your Sources of Iodine

Foods rich in iodine include:

- fish and seafood – clams, shrimps, haddock, halibut, oysters, salmon, sardines, tuna
- meat – beef, lamb, beef liver
- dairy foods – eggs, milk, butter, cream, cottage cheese, Cheddar cheese
- fruit and vegetables – pineapple, spinach, lettuce, green peppers, raisins, seaweed
- nuts and cereals – peanuts, wholemeal bread
- sea salt, iodized salt

Iodine has been known to be an essential component in our diet for over 150 years. A particularly rich source is marine products, such as fish, shellfish and seaweed, and it is found too in dairy produce, meat, poultry, grains and cereals. It is also used in the food industry in food colouring and dough conditioners.

Within the thyroid, iodine combines with other chemicals to produce T_3 and T_4. In fact, T_3 – the chemical name for triiodonine – is derived from the fact that it has three atoms of iodine, while T_4, is so called because it has four.

Lack of iodine causes the thyroid gland to form a swelling called a goitre, as it struggles to produce the hormones so vital to the body's processes. As long ago as the thirteenth century, physicians recommended burnt sponge, which is rich in iodine, as a treatment for goitre.

In the past, goitre caused by a lack of iodine in the soil was so common in the Pennines that it was known as Derbyshire neck. Even today, it's estimated that over 200 million people throughout the world suffer from iodine deficiency disorders, especially in areas far from the sea such as the Congo, the Andes, in Switzerland, around the Great Lakes in America, and in certain areas of Spain and Iran. There are estimated to be 1.5 million victims in the former Yugoslavia, and in parts of the Asian subcontinent nine out of ten of the population have goitre.

Strangely enough, too much iodine can be as harmful as too little, as in the case of the seaweed-eating Japanese fisherman who developed goitres as a result of consuming a staggering 10, 000 to 200, 000 micrograms a day! On a less grand scale, taking in too much iodine, for example in seaweed-based supplements such as kelp, or iodized cough sweets, can block production of the thyroid hormones and trigger a goitre.

Goitre Facts

A goitre may cause the whole of the thyroid to swell or be confined to just one clump of cells (a nodule). It may be symmetrical and form on both sides of the thyroid or affect just one side, and it may be soft, normal, firm or hard to the touch. If you have a goitre, the doctor will classify it according to size:

- small, if it can be felt but is not visible
- moderate, if it is visible but not large
- large, if it is visible and very obvious

There are many types of goitre, as you will see as you read on. Later on in the book, we shall see just how they are linked to different thyroid problems and what can be done about them.

Transporting Hormones

Virtually all the T_3 and T_4 in the body is carried around the bloodstream bound to two proteins. The remaining fraction is floating free in the blood. Once the two hormones have reached their destination, they are released from their protein binding and the T_4 is converted into the active T_3 form, ready for use by the cells. Free-floating T_3 doesn't have to be released from its binding and so is available for immediate use.

Certain factors, such as being on the Pill, can raise levels of protein in the blood, and in the past, thyroid tests were not always accurate because of the confusion this caused in the interpretation of results. Today's blood tests measure levels of the free-floating forms of T_3 and T_4 and these give a much more accurate indication of thyroid function.

When the Thyroid Gets Out of Balance

As we have seen, the hormones produced by the thyroid gland affect so many bodily processes and are needed to enable so many other hormones to work properly that it's hardly surprising that when something goes wrong your entire body is affected.

It has taken scientists almost 500 years to begin to unravel the mysteries of the thyroid. As long ago as the fifteenth century, anatomists had worked out the structure of the thyroid and recognized that it could become swollen, but it wasn't until the final decades of the nineteenth century that scientists began to work out exactly what was going wrong, a process that continues to this day.

In the past few years, interest has increasingly focused on the role the immune system has to play in thyroid disease, spurred at least in part by the hope that cracking the mystery of what causes the thyroid – a relatively easy organ to research – to turn against itself might illuminate the disease processes in less accessible autoimmune diseases like diabetes.

Chapter 3

HYPOTHYROIDISM: ALL SYSTEMS SLOW

Surveys show that women are five to ten times more likely to suffer from hypothyroidism – lack of thyroid hormones caused by an underactive thyroid gland – than men. In fact, it's estimated that 19 out of every 1000 women suffer from the condition, compared with just 1 in 1000 men. To cut the figures another way, according to one article in *Pulse*, a journal for British general practitioners, 10 out of every 1000 patients on the average GP's list will be on thyroid hormone replacement therapy because of an underactive thyroid.

Softly, Softly

Despite the figures, hypothyroidism is often missed or misdiagnosed. This is partly because it tends to sneak up insidiously and produce symptoms that are often confusing, such as depression and tiredness. Camille explains:

I noticed that my mental energy had gone right down, but I kept rationalizing my symptoms. The tiredness was dreadful but I persuaded myself it was because I was overdoing it. I kept saying to myself, 'If only I'd taken two weeks off at Christmas I wouldn't be feeling so tired'. It was only the hair loss that got me in for a test.

Clare, 39, who works as a local government officer recalls:

I just thought I was putting on weight. I put on two and a half stone in as many years. Yet, despite going to Weight Watchers and not cheating, I couldn't shift it. In retrospect there were other clues. I developed coarse skin, but because I'd had a baby and my hands were in and out of sterilizing solution, I just thought it was that. My periods were irregular and I was tired all the time, but I put that down to working and having a family. It was sheer vanity that drove me to the surgery in the end. My mother had had an overactive thyroid when she was pregnant with me and because of that I wondered if I had a thyroid problem.

My GP was brilliant and did a blood test which showed my thyroid was underactive.

Another sufferer, Jennifer, 38, a teacher who developed an underactive thyroid six years ago after the birth of her second child, remembers:

My energy levels fluctuated from day to day. I would start the week feeling fine, but by Tuesday I would be completely exhausted and have to take the day off. I managed to drag myself through Wednesday and Thursday, and Friday I had off. I would spend the weekend in bed. I was so depressed I would sometimes just lie there and cry. I had constant headaches and sore throats, my muscles ached, my nails were brittle, and I was always getting flu. I couldn't concentrate, my memory was appalling. I was so cold that even in the summer I had to take a hot-water bottle to bed. Our sex life went completely downhill. Despite all this, I couldn't get the doctor to take any notice. Eventually, I met a female doctor from my practice at a party, and she suggested I go in and have a thyroid test. It was the first mention of anything to do with the thyroid.

Sadly, Jennifer's experience is only too typical. Hypothyroidism is often referred to as myxoedema (from the Greek words 'myxa' for mucus and 'oedema' for swelling), though, strictly spreaking, this refers to the skin thickening that is often characteristic of the condition.

If you have hypothyroidism, your whole system slows down. The metabolism, running on near empty, is sluggish, so that what you eat is converted into energy more slowly and, as a result, you feel permanently cold. The smallest task becomes a supreme effort; you feel miserable, washed out and overwhelmed with fatigue. Another thing you may notice is that you are constantly going down with infections, as the lack of thyroid hormones takes its toll on your immune system, and cuts and bruises take a long time to heal, because of fragility of the blood vessels.

Appearance Matters

As the condition takes effect, the way you look may gradually change. Even though you have lost your appetite, the weight piles on. Your hair becomes dry, brittle and unmanageable and may drop out. Your skin, too, becomes dry, coarse and puffy. You may feel bloated – your waistband nips and your rings become too tight. Such thickening, which is known medically as myxoedema, is caused by the cells becoming leaky and depositing mucus underneath the skin. You may also develop a goitre, a clump of cells, which can cause the neck to increase in size. This is a result of the thyroid struggling to right itself. Alternatively, the thyroid may waste away, or atrophy. The swelling and thickening may also cause you to start snoring. And you may experience tingling and numbness in your hands, due to pressure on the nerves in the wrist caused by tissue swelling, a condition known as carpal tunnel syndrome. You may become pale and anaemic, and your complexion may take on a slightly yellowish tinge (due to an excess of the yellow pigment, beta-carotene in your blood).

Tired All the Time

Such physical changes can be extremely distressing, and they are compounded by the sheer exhaustion many hypothyroid sufferers experience, as Maggie, 34, who developed an underactive thyroid after the birth of her first child relates:

> *I put on an enormous amount of weight when I was expecting my first baby. After the baby was born, I felt totally paralysed for three days – I was so weak I could barely walk around. That slowly improved but I still felt slowed down, the way I imagine an old person must feel. I had no appetite, but even so the weight piled on. On one occasion I was actually ill with vomiting for three days and I still put on a pound! I was freezing cold all the time and had to keep the heating turned up high. My face was puffy, I looked as though I had been crying. My head felt as if it was full of cotton wool. I couldn't focus properly – if I looked at the TV and then tried to look at a newspaper, everything was blurred. I had noises in my ears. I slept very badly. I had pain and tingling in my hands that woke me up. I was also suffering from terrible constipation. I started losing my hair, but I just thought that was the normal hair loss that happens after pregnancy, but what was strange was that I didn't have to shave my legs or pluck my eyebrows. I felt as if my whole appearance was changing. The smallest task seemed enormous – I had trouble just walking to the corner of the road. Things came to a head when we went for a walk with some friends we were visiting. I was*

dragging myself along at my usual snail's pace, several yards behind. Being unable to keep up with the others really brought it home to me that it was more than just the after-effects of having had a baby; something was seriously wrong and I finally made an appointment with the doctor. My mother had an underactive thyroid, so because of that I was tested and discovered to be hypothyroid.

Feeling in a Fog

With this physical slowing down goes a mental sluggishness, depression and absent-mindedness. Sufferers may forget everyday events and there's an alarming time lag when you try to remember even familiar names or facts, described by many sufferers as feeling in a fog. Everything you attempt to do seems to take an age, and friends and family may comment that you have lost your get up and go.

In very severe cases, these mood changes and sense of muddle can lead on to more severe mental disturbance in which sufferers become out of touch with reality and develop paranoid feelings of persecution. Such symptoms, at one time cruelly described as 'myxoedematous madness', quickly disappear once treatment is given for the underactive thyroid.

The Senses

An underactive thyroid can affect your senses too, often as a result of tissue swelling. You may experience headaches and eyesight problems. You may become slightly deaf, or hear noises in the ears (tinnitus), your voice may become deep and husky, due to thickening of the vocal cords. Your digestive system may be impaired, your bowels slow down and you become constipated.

Menstrual Disturbances

Your periods may become heavier or stop altogether. If you are trying for a baby, you may have no success. And this may be at least partly because your sex life has ground to a halt. When everything is an effort, it can be hard to summon up the energy to make love, especially if you are feeling unattractive as a result of weight gain and other physical changes.

Affairs of the Heart

One of the more serious consequences of underactivity is heart problems, particularly in older women, who are more at risk of heart disease in the first place because of dwindling supplies of the hormone oestrogen after the menopause. You may notice you are short of breath when you walk fast, climb stairs or a hill. This is angina, caused by hardening of the arteries, when excess cholesterol is laid down in the bloodstream and begins to clog up the arteries, so not enough oxygen gets to the heart. Alternatively, you may experience calf pain (intermittent claudication), caused by furred arteries in the leg.

The reason for such symptoms is that your heart, like everything else, slows down. If you notice any of these symptoms, contact your doctor immediately.

The doctor will probably detect a low pulse rate (of under 60 beats a minute), which is abnormal in someone who is not athletic, together with high blood pressure and a raised blood cholesterol level.

Other Linked Illnesses

Early hypothyroidism may also be linked to anaemia, muscular disease and aches and pains in the joints (arthritis).

A Question of Depression

One of the most common features of hypothyroidism is depression. As a result, all too often, sufferers are misdiagnosed and referred to a psychologist, counsellor or psychiatrist. Dr Frank Tallis, writing in the *British Journal of Clinical Psychology* in 1993, observes that between 8 and 14 per cent of patients referred for 'depression' or some other emotional disorder are found to have some degree of hypothyroidism.

It can be hard to distinguish between them because the two illnesses share many common characteristics. Especially in milder cases of 'subclinical' disease, where depressed mood and lethargy may be the only symptoms, it's easy to be misdiagnosed. However, there are also some differences, as Table 3.1 shows, that, hopefully, will prompt the doctor to consider diagnosing hypothyroidism rather than depression.

Table 3.1 The similarities and differences between hypothyroidism and depression

Hypothyroidism	Depression
Weight gain	Weight loss
Loss of appetite	Appetite increase
Needing more sleep, tired all the time	Taking less sleep – insomnia, waking up early
Loss of sex drive and interest	Low self-esteem, guilt
Decreased concentration	
Poor memory	
Thinking slow, muddled	
Shared symptoms	
Miserable, feeling down	
Loss of interest or pleasure	

Unfortunately, if the doctor does misdiagnose you as suffering from depression and prescribes antidepressant drugs, Dr Tallis observes that you may actually get worse. Dwindling levels of thyroid hormones increase sensitivity to the side-effects of antidepressant drugs. So, if you are given them by mistake, you may experience the following symptoms:

- sleepiness
- dry mouth
- blurred vision
- constipation
- nausea
- difficulty passing water
- racing heart
- sweating
- trembling
- rashes

A Matter of Degree

Table 3.2 The symptoms of an underactive thyroid

What you might feel	What others might notice
Weight gain	Puffy face and dry, pale skin
Feeling cold	Swelling around the eyes
Weakness and muscular aches and pains	Coarseness of and loss of hair
Difficulty concentrating	Husky voice
Depression	Snoring
Difficult to manage hair, brittle nails	Slowness, loss of interest in former pleasures
Extreme tiredness and slowness	Deafness
Chest pain on exertion	
Constipation	
Period problems, infertility	**What the doctor may detect**
Loss of interest in sex	Doughy abdomen
Headaches, problems focusing	Goitre (swollen neck)
Sticky eyelids	Galactorrhoea (production of milk even if you aren't breastfeeding)
Slow healing, frequent infections	Delayed reflexes
Shortness of breath	Slowed pulse
Tingling in hands and feet	Carpal tunnel syndrome
Changes in skin pigmentation	Loss of muscle power
Muscle spasms	

Seeing all the symptoms of an underactive thyroid grouped together as they are in Table 3.2 may be somewhat alarming, but it does give you some idea of the vast number of ways in which your body can be affected. One thing is clear: the more symptoms you have, the more likely blood tests are to show abnormalities. In some countries, doctors have adopted a grading system for hypothyroid disorders, based on the number of symptoms together with the outcome of thyroid function tests, though this is not fully recognized in the UK (see Table 3.3).

Table 3.3 Grades of hypothyroidism

Severity of condition	What the the doctor might detect/ How you might feel
Grade 3 (subclinical)	Normal levels of thyroid hormones. Only very specialized tests would show abnormalities. Depression, tiredness, lethargy.
Grade 2	More definite feelings of being unwell with a few visible signs and symptoms. Blood tests show raised levels of TSH.
Grade 1	Swelling and facial changes and other visible signs and symptoms. Abnormal laboratory findings, such as raised TSH, low T_4, autoantibodies.

Causes of Hypothyroidism

So just why *does* the thyroid become underactive? The short answer is no one is quite sure (for a summary of the causes outlined below, see Table 3.4 on page 43). In 99 per cent of cases, something is the matter with the thyroid itself, and this is known as primary hypothyroidism. In the remaining 1 per cent, something is wrong with the pituitary or the hypothalamus, and this is called secondary hypothyroidism.

When the Body Turns Against Itself

The most common reason for the thyroid to become underactive is autoimmunity. This can cause a phenomenon known as spontaneous atrophic hypothyroidism, when the thyroid wastes away and shrinks, and also Hashimoto's disease (see below). It's been estimated that six times more women than men develop this, a result of the body literally turning against its own tissues as if they were foreign and trying to destroy them with antibodies. And 15 times more women than men suffer from Hashimoto's disease. Collectively, the two are known as autoimmune hypothyroid disorder and account for around 45 per cent of hypothyroid cases.

But, why should a mechanism designed to protect the body and keep it healthy go so dramatically wrong? The experts can't agree on whether autoantibodies are a cause or an effect of the autoimmune process. There is much debate, too, over whether or not the process is due to the alteration of normal body proteins or autoantibodies that are normally present only beginning to cause trouble because the mechanisms for keeping them in check break down, as a result of factors such as infection or as we get older.

The Body's Defence System

To understand how the body can turn against itself in this way it's necessary to understand a bit about the way the immune system works.

The body's defence system is extremely complicated, but many of its actions depend on certain types of white blood cells, known as lymphocytes, which produce immunity, or resistance to disease. Each one of our body's cells is imprinted with a code that enables the lymphocytes to recognize them as belonging to 'self' and thus leave them alone. If the body is attacked by invaders, such as bacteria or viruses, the immune system recognizes them as foreign and sends lymphocytes, known as T-lymphocytes, to attack and destroy them by producing antibodies. T-lymphocytes are involved in both switching on and switching off the immune system. When you get better, the body retains a 'memory' of the invader, which is stored in special memory cells called B-lymphocytes. The next time the same invader threatens, these memory cells recognize it, form antibodies, and the T-lymphocytes rush in for the kill.

The Enemy Within

Normally, either before or soon after birth, the T-lymphocytes are programmed to recognize and distinguish the body's own tissues from invaders. However, for some reason, some cells may escape recognition and, later in life, they may be discovered by the T-lymphocytes and attacked. Sometimes certain body proteins are altered by infection, drugs, pollution and other factors with the result that the T-lymphocytes no longer recognize them as belonging and form antibodies against them. These 'self' antibodies are known as autoantibodies – from the word 'auto', which means 'self'.

Autoantibodies can attack almost any of the body's tissues or organs, causing a range of autoimmune diseases in which the tissues become inflamed and are gradually destroyed. It can happen in the kidneys (causing glomerulonephritis), the joints (causing rheumatoid arthritis), the adrenal glands (causing Addison's disease), the stomach (causing pernicious anaemia, due to a damaged ability to absorb the vitamin B_{12}), the pancreas (causing diabetes) and, of course, the thyroid.

Once the body has turned against one organ or tissue, it is more prone to do the same against another. Hence, suffering from any one of these diseases puts you at an increased risk of also suffering one of the others. For this reason, if you have an autoimmune thyroid disorder, the doctor should be on the lookout for other autoimmune problems.

When the Key Doesn't Fit

In one in five of those with autoimmune hypothyroidism, the antibodies produced block TSH receptors on the surface of thyroid cells. TSH, if you remember, is the thyroid stimulating hormone produced by the pituitary, which triggers the thyroid into action. When this happens, the TSH is produced normally but is unable to stimulate the thyroid to produce its hormones. It's a bit like trying to unlock a door and finding the keyhole blocked.

Antibody Action

In other cases, the autoantibodies search out and destroy the thyroid cells. When this happens, lymphocytes may completely or partially replace the normal thyroid tissue, causing severe inflammation – a process known as infiltration. This inflammation is known as thyroiditis. Sometimes it is caused by a virus, but often it is caused by the presence of autoimmune antibodies. In its viral form it may start with a swollen, tender thyroid, a bit like when you are going down with a cold.

The Family Factor

The tendency for autoimmune problems to run in families offers one clue as to the underlying cause. It suggests that a faulty gene or genes may be to blame for preventing the body from protecting itself against 'self attack'. Defective genes may also prevent T_3 and T_4 from trapping the necessary atoms of iodine or be responsible for faulty synthesis of the carrier protein in which the hormones travel around the bloodstream.

Lack of Iodine

There are of course other causes of hypothyroidism. In the past, and in some parts of the world even today, as we have seen, one of the main ones was quite simply a shortage of iodine in the diet. However, in the West, with the availability of iodized salt, this is far less likely to be the problem.

Medical Treatment

Ironically, in one in three cases, the gland becomes underactive as a result of medical treatments for overactivity, such as after taking the drug carbimazole or having radioactive iodine treatment or thyroid surgery. If you have had your thyroid completely removed (total thyroidectomy), of course the body will no longer be able to produce thyroid hormones. However, even if you have only had *part* of the thyroid removed (subtotal/partial thyroidectomy), you stand a one in three or four chance of developing underactivity within ten years of the operation. Other medical triggers include drugs containing iodine (iodides), such as some cough remedies, and lithium, which is used to treat manic depression.

Pregnancy and Childbirth

The thyroid also tends to slow down during pregnancy and problems often start after childbirth, or even sometimes a miscarriage. Chapter 6 deals with this important cause of thyroid underactivity.

Congenital (Problems Present from Birth)

About 1 in 5000 babies are born with an underactive thyroid. Sometimes the gland has become inflamed in the womb (*in utero* thyroiditis), but the most common reason is that it fails to develop altogether – a problem more likely to affect baby girls than baby boys, which, again, suggests a genetic or hormonal connection.

In the past, such individuals were termed cretins. But, as this word has come to be used as a term of abuse, it has tended to fall out of use. The problem often tends to run in families, though the pattern of inheritance is such that it doesn't simply pass down from one generation to the next. Intriguingly, the mothers of such babies are more likely than average to have autoimmune thyroiditis.

Some newborn babies have a goitre (endemic goitre), due to faulty synthesis of hormones, caused by a metabolic disorder.

Hashimoto's Disease

In adults, a condition called Hashimoto's disease is the most common cause of autoimmune hypothyroidism. The condition – sometimes called Hashimoto's thyroiditis because it involves inflammation of the thyroid – strikes five times more women than men.

At first, although you may not feel ill, you may develop a small goitre. As time goes on, this may become tender and feel uncomfortable when you swallow. Curiously, when the disease first develops, you may actually develop the symptoms of an *overactive* thyroid – you may lose weight, your heart pounds, your digestive system goes into overdrive, you have diarrhoea, you cannot stand the heat, and your eyes may become wide and staring. Such problems are only temporary, however, and as the disease progresses, the thyroid becomes less and less active and the typical signs and symptoms of hypothyroidism set in.

Thyroid Cancer

Very, very occasionally, the cause of the underactivity may be cancer. Although the word 'cancer' tends to strike terror into anyone's heart, do bear in mind that thyroid cancer is extremely rare. It accounts for just 1 per cent of all cases of cancer, and is one of the most curable types of cancer. It's not known exactly why it develops, though exposure to radioactive fallout is one risk factor, as the hugely increased incidence of thyroid cancer in the children living around the Chernobyl area has shown.

Secondary Hypothyroidism

In a few cases, the problem lies not in your thyroid at all, but in the gland that controls it, the pituitary, or the body's overall control centre, the hypothalamus in the brain. Scientists are only just beginning to understand all the things that can go wrong at this level, but, it is thought, in some cases, that abnormalities in the production of TRH (thyrotropin releasing hormone) could be linked to interferences in the transmission of messages between nerve cells and hormones.

Problems of pituitary development or the development of tumours or cysts may have a knock-on effect on the production of thyroid hormones. In other cases, the pituitary appears to secrete an inactive form of TSH, which is unable to bind on to receptors in the thyroid.

Table 3.4 Why is my thyroid underactive?

Primary hypothyroidism
Thyroiditis (inflammation of the thyroid) as a result of: • Hashimoto's disease • viral infection
Medical treatment: • total removal of the thyroid (thyroidectomy) • partial removal of the thyroid (thyroidectomy) • radioactive iodine treatment
Drug induced, for example: • carbimazole (for an overactive thyroid) • iodine compounds • lithium used to treat manic depression
After childbirth See Chapter 6
Thyroid cancer
Present at birth (congenital): • absence of thyroid • abnormal development of thyroid • metabolic defect
Secondary hypothyroidism
Pituitary problems Hypothalamic problems

Chapter 4

HYPERTHYROIDISM: LIFE IN THE FAST LANE

Overproduction of thyroid hormones, hyperthyroidism (or thyrotoxicosis, as it's sometimes called) is caused by the thyroid becoming overactive. The condition is usually much easier to spot than hypothyroidism, partly because it has such obvious effects mentally and physically (for a summary of these, see Table 4.1). An estimated 1 in 50 people suffer from it and 9 out of 10 of these are women.

Hyperthyroidism is the reverse side of the hypothyroidism coin. Where an underactive thyroid slows your body down, an overactive one causes the metabolism to race. Jan, 42, who sufferers from Graves' disease, one of the most common types of hyperthyroidism, has the following to say about her symptoms, which are typical of this kind of thryroid problem:

I'd had a lot of trouble in my marriage and a lot of stress generally after I left. The first thing I noticed was that I was full of energy. I couldn't sit still, I had to be working, working out, cooking or doing something with the kids all the time. I started to drink to try and slow myself down. As time went on, I couldn't sit down long enough to think and I became totally exhausted. My muscles

Table 4.1 A case of overactivity

What you may feel	What others may notice
Increased sweating	Mood changes
Sensation of warmth	Talkativeness
Oversensitivity to heat	Agitation
Warm, moist palms	Appearance changes, such as swollen neck, staring eyes
Nervousness, anxiety, excitability	Weight loss
Insomnia/racing thoughts	Shakiness/trembling
Palpitations	Skin changes
Weight loss	**What the doctor may detect**
Weak, less defined muscles (wasting)	Tremor
Increased appetite	Low blood pressure
Period problems, such as no periods, longer or shorter cycle	Fast pulse
Eye complaints	Irregular heartbeat (atrial fibrilation)
Dry, thin skin that flushes easily, hair loss	Brisk reflexes
Goitre	
Increased sex drive	
Loss of muscle strength	
Staring eyes	

started to waste, even though I was exercising so much. My periods stopped. I had bouts of breathlessness, which were diagnosed as asthma. I couldn't think straight, my mind was so overactive. I felt as if my head was full of twittering sparrows and I had what I can only describe as an 'electrical buzzing' in my head.

Other sufferers talk of feeling constantly hot and sweaty, stripping off and throwing windows open, even on cold days. They may also develop diarrhoea, a symptom so common that hyperthyroidism is frequently picked up in gastroenterology clinics.

As Jan's experience illustrates, when the thyroid becomes overactive, the body burns up energy at a tremendous rate. Sufferers eat like elephants without putting on any weight. In fact, more often than not, they lose it at an alarming rate.

Some sufferers also experience a raging thirst and pass large amounts of urine, in a way very similar to diabetics. In one of the few studies of this phenomenon carried out in 1991, a team of doctors from Leeds and Newcastle in the UK tested seven women and one man who had recently been diagnosed as suffering from hyperthyroidism. Their findings suggest that the overactivity of the thyroid somehow disturbs centres in the brain that control the thirst threshold. This disturbance seems in turn to be linked to the secretion of vasopressin, a hormone that causes the kidneys to retain water and prevents excessive water being passed as urine.

Intriguingly, the researchers suggest that the phenomenon may be linked to anxiety, another well-known feature of hyperthyroidism. The link is via the production of a protein called angiotensin II, which is involved in stimulating the adrenal glands to produce a hormone that boosts blood pressure.

Certainly anyone who has been around someone with an overactive thyroid can't fail to notice their boundless nervous energy. Sufferers pace around like caged lions, talking nineteen to the dozen, yet they are unable to muster any concentration. Their tremendous energy never flags for a second, even at bedtime, as Louise, 38, recalls:

> *I couldn't settle for the jumble of racing thoughts that were flying around my brain. My sex drive increased, too – I wouldn't leave my husband alone.*

Louise's experience echoes that of other sufferers, and it is thought to occur because of the increased turnover of male sex hormones, androgens, which control the libido, and which are converted into the female hormone, oestrogen, in the body.

Mood Swings

The hyperthyroid sufferer's moods often swing wildly from euphoria to depression. And just as hypothyroid symptoms are often mistakenly attributed to depression, anxiety may be seen as a cause rather than an effect of the problem. Again, as sufferers with an underactive thyroid find, it's not unheard of for sufferers to be referred to a psychiatrist before it's realized that the cause of the problem is an overactive thyroid.

Appearance Matters Too

An overactive thyroid affects appearance. The skin becomes thin, hot, pink and moist. Sufferers tend to flush easily, and the blush extends down the neck and on to the chest. Their palms are red and sweaty, their hair becomes fine and flyaway and may start to fall out, and the nails become thin and flaky.

Some sufferers develop thyrotoxic tremor – a constant fine trembling that is most noticeable if you stretch out your hands. This is thought to be due to oversensitivity to the stress hormone, adrenalin. Maria, 35, a former nursery nurse, whose thyroid became overactive two years ago, recalls that this tremor was the first thing she noticed when her thyroid became overactive:

> *I first became aware of the problem when I noticed that I wasn't able to hold my camera steady (I'm a freelance photographer). I couldn't hold a pen straight to write either, and I started having palpitations. My heart beat so fast that on one occasion I was convinced that I was going to have a heart attack. I was losing weight*

rapidly: I went from my usual 8½ to 9 stone to 7½, even though I was eating like a pig. And I was irritable and bad-tempered.

Heart and Bone

The palpitations Maria describes are another common feature, caused by overactivity of the heart muscle, which leads to an acceleration of the pulse rate, palpitations and an irregular heartbeat. Older women who develop hyperthyroidism are particularly prone to such problems, which has led more than the occasional sufferer to have been misdiagnosed as having suffered a heart attack.

Breathlessness is another common symptom and this, too, is sometimes misdiagnosed, this time as asthma or bronchitis. The slightest exertion can bring on an attack. A side-effect of this is that untreated overactivity can actually damage the heart.

Overactivity of the thyroid can also disturb the body's calcium balance, which can lead to less of this important mineral being laid down in the bones, increasing the risk of osteoporosis.

Weakness, caused by muscle wastage, is another problem for about half of all sufferers. As Sarah remembers:

I am a marathon runner, but I just couldn't run at all. If I got down on the floor, someone had to help me up.

In a few very rare cases, particularly for some reason in those of Oriental background, sufferers experience periodic paralysis – attacks of paralysis caused the body's inability to keep a constant concentration of potassium in the blood.

The Goitre Connection

As with an underactive thyroid, an overactive one can also cause a goitre. This can vary from a slight fullness in the neck to a swelling so pronounced that sufferers have trouble fastening close-fitting necklaces and are no longer able to do up the top button on shirts and blouses.

Most sufferers have something called a smooth, soft goitre. As the name suggests, it is smooth in texture and soft to the touch. It is also rich in blood vessels, so if you place your fingers on it you may even be able to feel the blood rushing through it. If the doctor listens to it through a stethoscope, it may be possible to hear the blood surging turbulently through the vessels, a noise known as a 'thyroid bruit' (a bruit is the sound made in the heart, arteries or veins when blood circulation flows at an abnormal speed).

Eye Changes

One of the most tell-tale signs of thyroid overactivity are changes in the eyes. You may notice any of the following:

- staring appearance
- white of eyes visible between iris and lower lid
- white of eyes visible above iris and upper lid
- swelling of tissues around the eye, causing bags under the eyes and swollen eyelids
- problems with focusing or double vision

Although bulging eyes are one of the features people tend to associate with thyroid problems, such eye changes are not a simple matter of cause and effect. In fact, only around 1 in 20 hyperthyroidism sufferers actually develops severe eye problems. They tend to be linked to particular types of hyperthyroidism, especially the autoimmune type. Others may develop some eye symptoms that disappear once the thyroid problem is brought under control, and it's even possible to develop eye problems without there being any abnormality of the thyroid. Eye problems occurring in the absence of thyroid disease are known as ophthalmic Graves' disease (all these topics are covered in the next chapter).

Sufferers who develop eye changes are also prone to developing patches of slightly reddened, thickened skin on the lower legs. The hair on these areas tends to become coarser, too. This condition, known as pretibial myxoedema, can sometimes develop years after an attack of hyperthyroidism. The eye changes, together with the other physical aspects of an overactive thyroid, can be some of the worst effects to bear, as Jan recalls:

> *I developed brown circles under my eyes, and my eyelids started to swell. I didn't really notice it myself because I don't look in the mirror much, but other people kept commenting on it. My hair started to fall out. I looked like a gargoyle with horrible bulgy eyes and virtually no hair. People thought I was on drugs. Eventually I became so self-conscious that I avoided going out. I thought I was going insane. Eventually, I had a thyroid test at the hospital, which was so high they sent me straight to the doctor's surgery – within half an hour I was on antithyroid drugs.*

The Causes of Hyperthyroidism

Table 4.2 Causes of overactivity

Common causes
Graves' disease
Toxic multinodular goitre (Plummer's disease)
Toxic adenoma
Rarer causes
Excess iodine
After childbirth (post-partum thyroiditis)
Silent thyroiditis
Addiction to thyroid hormones (thyrotoxicosis factitia)
Problems with the pituitary

Graves' Disease

The most common cause of all these symptoms – that is, in eight out of ten cases – is a condition known as Graves' disease. Like Hashimoto's disease, this is an autoimmune condition, caused by the immune system reacting as if its own tissue were foreign. It tends to run in families and is linked to other autoimmune diseases. In fact, Graves' and Hashimoto's often cluster in families, leading doctors to suspect that a common gene or group of genes is responsible. It's most common between the ages of 20 and 40, but it can strike girls as young as 5 and, very occasionally, the babies of sufferers.

The man who gave his name to the illness was an Irish doctor, Robert James Graves, who worked at the Meath Hospital in Dublin. In 1835, he published a paper describing the typical symptoms of overactive thyroid together with goitre in six recently pregnant women, underlining the connection with pregnancy, which we shall examine more closely in Chapter 6. The condition is known as Graves' disease in the UK and the US, but in Europe it is often called Basedow's disease, after another doctor, Carl A. von Basedow, a private practitioner in Germany, who described the illness in three women in 1840.

When the Immune System Goes Wrong

So just what triggers the body to turn against itself in Graves' disease? Frustratingly, once again doctors still haven't found the answer, but one theory is that it is due to a genetically determined fault in the functioning of suppressor T cells, which inhibit the activity of other cells involved in the immune response. As a result, antibodies against areas of the membrane of the thyroid cell containing TSH receptors are produced, which cause the thyroid gland to grow and overproduce T_3 and T_4.

One possible culprit could be an abnormal antibody, known as long-acting thyroid stimulator (LATS) – believed to be responsible for the action of TSH receptor cells in the thyroid – which has been found in 50 to 60 per cent of sufferers with Graves' disease.

Another potential candidate could be another antibody called LATS-protector, found in nine out of ten sufferers, which blocks TSH from binding to the membrane of the thyroid cell.

But where do the antibodies come from? One theory is that the thyroid cells themselves possess faulty TSH receptors. These trigger the production of thyroid-stimulating antibodies and it's this that stimulates overproduction of thyroid hormones. Another theory is that there is a faulty immune mechanism, in that the body fails to recognize the antibodies as being potentially harmful or it tries to quell their action but cannot do so in time.

Could There be a Food Poisoning Connection?

One of the most intriguing suggestions, described by US surgeon Mr David V. Feliciano in the *American Journal of Surgery* in November 1992, is that the process is sparked off by infection with a food poisoning bug known as *Yersinia enterocolitica*. The bug, a distant relative of the plague bug, is fond of milk and causes stomach pain, fever, diarrhoea and a sore throat. One of its nastier attributes is that it grows happily in normal fridge temperatures.

Yersinia has a special binding site – a place where TSH locks on – for TSH in its cell membrane. Thus, if someone, at risk of Graves' disease because of a genetic predisposition, say, contracts yersinia, it's suggested that 'antibodies that would arise might cross-react with TSH-binding sites in the membrane of the human thyroid cell' – a case of mistaken identity that could spark an autoimmune reaction.

Although the theory hasn't been proved, backing comes from the fact that sufferers from both Graves' and Hashimoto's disease have been found to have clumps of antibodies against yersinia in their bloodstream.

Is Stress to Blame?

In the past few years, there's been increasing evidence that, in a number of illnesses, the immune system is weakened by negative mental states such as fear, tension, overwork, anxiety and exhaustion – in a word, stress. So, could stress be responsible for Graves' disease?

According to Feliciano, in the nineteenth century, doctors observed that Graves' disease often followed on from a period of severe emotional stress, a frightening episode or 'actual or threatened separation from an individual upon whom the patient is emotionally dependent'.

The nineteenth-century physician Caleb Hillier Parry, who practised in Bath and whose description of the symptoms of the disease predate those of Graves himself by 10 years, was one of the first to consider the stress connection:

> *Elizabeth S., aged 21, was thrown out of a wheelchair in coming fast down hill, 28th April last, and very much frightened, though not much hurt. From this time she has been subject to palpitation of the heart, and various nervous affections. About a fortnight after this period she began to observe a swelling of the thyroid gland.*

In Norway and Denmark, the incidence of hyperthyroidism increased during the first years of the Second World War. In their book, *Thyroid Disease: The Facts,* doctors Bayliss and Tunbridge mention some intriguing research showing a significant rise in the incidence of Graves' disease in Northern Ireland since the start of political troubles in 1968.

The trouble is that many of the accounts of the link between stress and Graves' disease were anecdotal, and earlier studies have been criticized for not being carried out under scientific conditions, with a proper control group. What's more, in some cases, the diagnosis of Graves' disease was questionable. As a result, many doctors dismissed any connection between stress and Graves' disease – until recently.

In 1991, a team of Swedish researchers from Uppsala chose 208 newly diagnosed Graves' disease sufferers and compared them with a control group of 372 people. They had to answer a detailed questionnaire about their lifestyles and personality, together with details about any significant life events, such as divorce, that had occurred during the previous year.

Astonishingly, the Graves' disease sufferers were found to be far more likely to have suffered an unhappy event. The death of a close relative or friend was reported by 15 per cent of the Graves' disease sufferers, but only 10 per cent of the controls. The disease was also more likely to strike those who were divorced, and who were less happy with their jobs than the control group – all suggesting that long-term anxiety, unhappiness and other negative feelings could be a factor.

The researchers, writing in the *Lancet*, also observed that those with Graves' disease were more likely to have had more than five minor infections, such as cystitis and colds, in the previous year. Given that going down with infections is a sign that your immune defences are lowered, could it be that in Graves' disease stress somehow damages the immune system, causing it turn against itself? Is it that Graves' disease sufferers are more susceptible to minor infections? Or is it simply that if you are feeling unwell anyway you are more likely to notice such infections? Such questions remain unanswered.

Of course, all this doesn't prove that stress is to blame for triggering Graves' disease, but it does suggest it could be an important factor. One of the difficulties is that the disease creeps up insidiously so it's not entirely clear whether the stressful events happened before or after the true onset of the disease. And whether the link is a physical one or you are simply more likely to notice physical complaints that you ignored during a period of stress remains to be discovered. Whatever the answer, the research certainly suggests a line worth pursuing.

Is It Really Graves' Disease?

Graves' disease has been called the 'great masquerader' because it doesn't always produce the typical symptoms of an overactive thyroid. Instead of being agitated and overactive, some suffers become lethargic and passive, unable to do anything but lie in bed all day. Patricia, 34, who was diagnosed with an overactive thyroid two years ago, recalls:

> *In the past I was always a very active person. I love sports and would be out playing tennis or squash or doing aerobics four or five times a week. A couple of years ago I began to feel completely worn out, I started to put on weight. My muscles ached all over and I felt*

fluey. I really strugged to get through each day. I was backwards and forwards to the doctor for about six months, but each time I was diagnosed as having flu or a virus.

My mother suffers from an underactive thyroid, so when my neck began to swell I asked the doctor if I could have a thyroid problem. He said, 'No'. He thought it was a problem with my ears, because my job involves a lot of flying abroad. Eventually I saw an ENT specialist who felt my neck and said, 'Are you being treated for your thyroid problem?' Two days later I was back at the hospital having tests, which showed I had an overactive thyroid. My symptoms weren't at all typical, which I guess is why it took so long to get a diagnosis.

Such symptoms tend to be more common in older women who develop an overactive thyroid, and such sufferers may be labelled depressive or thought to be suffering from a hidden cancer. This type of hyperthyroidism – known as apathetic thyrotoxicosis – can be particularly tricky for a doctor to detect as the true cause of the condition is masked, and this can lead to delays in diagnosis. But it is important to get it diagnosed as such apathy is a sign that the overactive metabolism has reached the point of burn-out and urgent treatment is needed to bring the thyroid under control.

Thyroid Nodules

Graves' disease isn't the only reason for the thyroid becoming overactive. In some cases, the fault lies not in the thyroid itself, but in abnormal stimulation of the gland, which causes it to produce too many hormones, creating a lumpy swelling.

For 15 per cent of sufferers, an overactive thyroid causes an existing goitre to become lumpy and irregular, or nodular. A nodular goitre may be caused by a shortage or excess of iodine in the diet or in certain drugs, such as cough medicines or food supplements. Sometimes it's because of erratic overstimulation of part of the thyroid by TSH, the thyroid hormone produced by the pituitary. Although it's possible for the thyroid to operate normally in such cases, as time goes on, the nodules may become overactive. This form of overactivity, known as toxic multinodular goitre or sometimes as Plummer's disease, tends to be particularly common in older women. If the goitre becomes particularly large, it can cause discomfort in the neck and may even occasionally interfere with breathing or swallowing.

In a further 5 per cent of cases, overactivity is caused by a single nodule becoming overactive, a condition known as toxic adenoma, or a hot nodule (an adenoma is a benign, non-cancerous lump). This, too, is more common in middle age and later life. The overactivity may occur as the nodule increases in size and, again, it may be sparked off by increased iodine intake.

Is It Cancer?

Being told you have a lump is always worrying as most of us tend to associate such lumps with cancer. However, nodules of the type described are extremely unlikely to be cancerous (malignant). The doctor may want to make completely sure by doing an ultrasound scan to determine the composition of the nodule, seeing whether it is filled with fluid (a cyst) or solid. If it is solid, a few cells may be withdrawn with a needle (fine needle biopsy) to check for possible malignant changes. So-called 'cold' nodules are more likely to be cancerous.

Other Reasons for Overactivity

There are several other causes of hyperthyroidism. These include the following.

- Excess iodine *As we've seen, too much iodine can be as harmful to the thyroid as too little, particularly if you already have an existing thyroid problem. In this case, severe hyperthyroidism can result, a condition known as Jod-Basedow disease.*

- Childbirth *Post-partum thyroiditis occurs in around 5 out of every 100 women after having a baby and is dealt with more fully in Chapter 6.*

- The hamburger syndrome *Inflammation of the thyroid that causes no pain or discomfort to the thyroid gland, which has led to it being termed 'silent'. Thyroid enlargement may be modest and there are no effects on the eyes. It's a self-limiting condition that normally lasts for a few months. Although it's rarely reported in the UK, in the US some cases have been found to result from eating too many hamburgers contaminated with thyroid tissue from the neck muscles of cows.*

- The thyroxine 'high' *Thyroid hormones act as stimulants. Some sufferers treated with thyroxine for an underactive thyroid enjoy the sense of increased energy and well-being so much that they become addicted to it and start to 'overdose' – a condition known as thyrotoxicosis factitia – which causes the thyroid to become overactive. Doctors tend to say this isn't very common, but the fact is that no one knows just how many women take that little bit extra, sometimes to help control their weight. Needless to say, it's a dangerous practice as an overactive thyroid is much more difficult to treat than an underactive one.*

- Problems with the pituitary *Occasionally, the pituitary produces too much TSH, which overstimulates the thyroid. Although rare, this form of hyperthyroidism is being recognized more frequently now that more sensitive blood tests are available. Very occasionally, the raised TSH may be caused by a pituitary tumour, which can be detected by a skull X-ray or CT scan.*

Chapter 5

The Eyes Have It: Dealing with Thyroid Eye Problems

One of the most distressing aspects of thyroid disease is undoubtedly the development of the potentially disfiguring and sight-threatening eye problems known as Graves' ophthalmopathy. As the name suggests, such problems are particularly likely to be linked to Graves' disease, with up to half of all sufferers having obviously protruding eyes. However, the advent of sophisticated scanning techniques, which allow doctors to build up cross-sectional pictures of the inside of the body, has revealed that, in fact, the disease has some effect on the eyes of practically all sufferers, even though this may not be immediately noticeable.

Far too little is known about the causes of such problems and, so far, no way of preventing them has been found. Given that the same disturbances can sometimes occur in people whose thyroid function is apparently perfectly normal and also in Hashimoto's disease sufferers, some doctors, especially in the US, prefer to use the terms 'thyroid-associated ophthalmopathy' or 'dysthyroid orbitopathy' to describe these eye problems. One result of the lack of understanding of thyroid eye problems is that, at present, the choice of treatments is sadly still somewhat limited.

Signs and Symptoms

The problems can involve all the components of your eyes. Friends or relatives may be the first to notice and comment on the characteristically bulging eyeballs that medically are known as proptosis or sometimes exophthalmos, which results in the staring appearance most of us recognize as being part of this condition (see Figure 5.1).

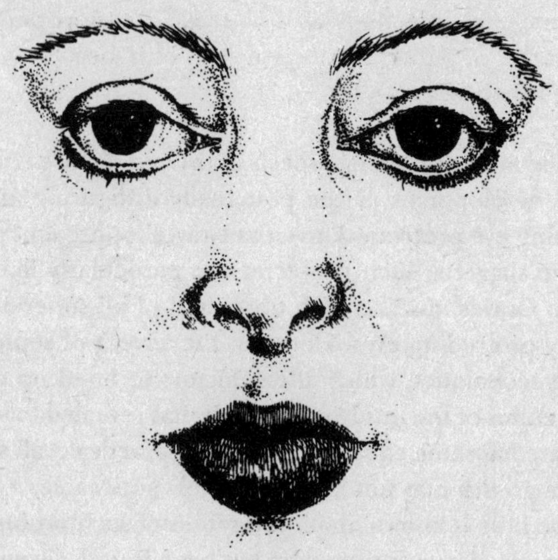

***Figure 5.1** Proptosis, or, exophthalmos – a typical eye symptom in Graves' disease. The eyes protrude and the white shell of the eye (sclera) is visible between the lower lid and cornea (the invisible circle of tissue that covers the iris and pupil).*

To understand how this happens, it helps to understand a little about the anatomy of the eye. Our eyeballs lie enclosed in pear-shaped bony sockets known as the orbits, each lined with protective pads of fat, connective tissue, blood vessels, muscles, nerves and the lacrimal glands, where tears are formed. If these tissues become swollen, as a result of inflammation, the eyeball will be pushed forwards. Both eyes are usually affected, but occasionally one protrudes more than the other.

You may notice that your eyes are puffy, with bags under the eyes, a tendency to water, redness and that they are bloodshot at the outer corners (see Figure 5.2). You may experience a deep pressure within the eye socket and feel a burning or gritty sensation, a result of your eyes being less protected by the eyelids from dust, wind and infection. And you may develop photophobia (intolerance of light), so that you can only bear to go outside wearing sunglasses.

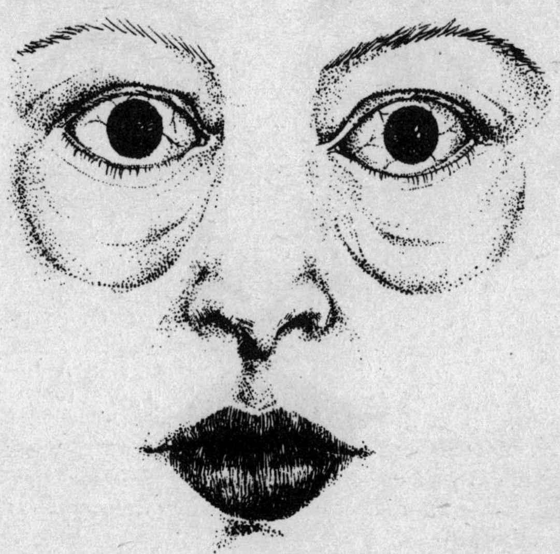

***Figure* 5.2** *Peri-orbital swelling – swelling above and below the eyes – occurs in Graves' disease.*

At the same time, as a result of the inflammation, the muscles are unable to work effectively – a condition known medically as ophthalmoplegia, which, in turn, can cause double vision (see Figure 5.3). You may also experience a phenomenon called lid lag, which is when the upper lids are slow to follow the downward movement of your eyes when you look down. Very occasionally, the increased pressure within the eye socket also affects the optic nerve, leading to blurred vision and a dulling of colour perception. In the past, when such problems were less likely to be detected in time, some sufferers even went blind. Fortunately this is very unlikely to happen today as there are more sophisticated ways of detecting eye disease.

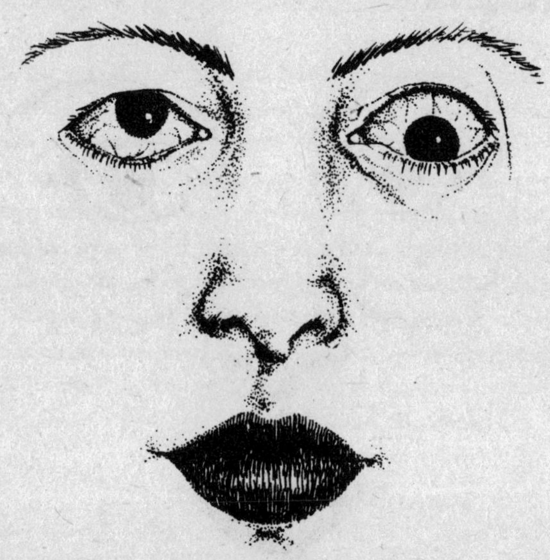

***Figure 5.3** Ophthalmoplegia, a weakness or paralysis of the muscles controlling eye movement affects upward and outward gaze, may cause double vision.*

Just to make things even more confusing, the changes linked to Graves' disease can come on as much as a year and a half before or after the development of other symptoms of overactivity, and do so in eight out of ten cases. Most often, though, the eye symptoms develop at the same time as other symptoms. Lucy's story is fairly typical:

> *I have Graves' disease, which presented as diarrhoea. At first, the doctors thought there was something wrong with my gut, and I was referred to the hospital for tests. Meantime, my eyes felt really sore and gritty. I was given steroids for the gut problems, so the eyes didn't bother me for a while, but eventually, when I did get diagnosed with Graves', I stopped taking them, and then my eyes did start to really play up.*
>
> *At first my eyes were very sore and red and other people noticed they were changing in appearance, though I was unaware of it to begin with. They became very sore and swollen with an incredible feeling of pressure. Then I started to find it hard to move the muscles, so I have to turn my whole head to look left and right. My upper lids are very swollen and puffy, I had some lid lag and straining and I had horrible bags under my eyes, though that is better now. It is a horrible thing to happen. One of the worst things was that people who hadn't seen me for some time wouldn't recognize me. At present they are waiting for the overactivity to settle down, but eventually I may have plastic surgery.*

Other Physical Changes

Interestingly, one of the least common symptoms of Graves' disease, pretibial dermopathy, which is when red, thickened patches of skin appear, particularly on the front of the lower legs and sometimes elsewhere, is found in about one in ten sufferers with severe ophthalmopathy. However, in a review which appeared in the *New England Journal of Medicine*, endocrinologists Drs Rebecca

S. Bahn and Armin E. Heufelder of the Mayo Clinic describe how subtle abnormalities in the skin cells that produce no obvious swelling or thickening have been detected in seven out of ten Graves' disease sufferers by taking a biopsy (a small shaving of skin). The doctors point out that, when analysed, the skin cells involved in pretibial dermopathy and connective tissue cells from the orbit show close similarities, suggesting a common underlying cause.

Eye Problems Not Due to Graves' Disease

Not all eye symptoms brought on by overactivity of the thyroid are due to Graves' disease, and it's important to distinguish between the two groups of problems because hyperthyroid eye disease *not* caused by Graves' disease tends to be much easier to treat.

The main signs of this second group are a condition known as lid retraction, in which the upper eyelids are pulled upwards, exposing more of the whites of your eyes than normal, producing a staring appearance, which mimics proptosis (see Figure 5.4). Wateriness, discomfort, redness and intolerance of light can also accompany this apparent proptosis, but tend to subside once the overactive thyroid is brought under control. Unfortunately, the eye changes linked to Graves' disease are often more troublesome than this and can take some time to settle.

What Causes Graves' Ophthalmopathy?

Like the thyroid overactivity caused by Graves' disease itself, Graves' ophthalmopathy is now known to be a result of the body turning against itself, a tendency that, like other autoimmune conditions, tends to be inherited. However, the precise mechanism involved remains a subject of intense debate, though doctors agree that both environmental and genetic factors operating

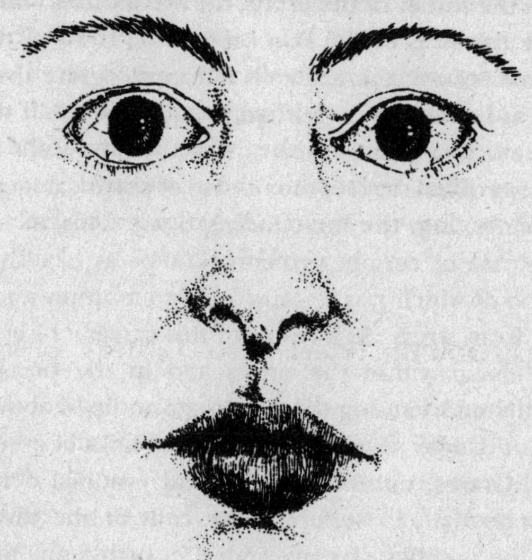

Figure 5.4 Lid retraction – a spasm of the upper eyelid pulls it up, causing the whites of the eyes to be visible above the cornea.

on the immune system almost certainly play a part.

The most characteristic feature of eye problems linked to Graves' disease is enlargement of the muscles that move the eyes and of the fatty connective tissue within the orbits caused by inflammation. It's this that causes the eyeballs to bulge forwards. Doctors don't understand exactly what triggers the inflammation, but one clue comes from the discovery that some Graves' ophthalmopathy sufferers have antibodies in their bloodstream directed towards eye muscle or connective tissue. The tissue of their orbits, too, has been found to contain antibodies that are poisonous to eye muscle cells.

In an article that appeared in the *Annual Review of Medicine,* 1992, US endocrinologists Judy A. Carter and Robert D. Utiger suggest that the inflammatory process starts with the gathering of T-lymphocytes (white blood cells involved in the immune reaction) within the tissues of the orbits, the eye muscles and the tear glands, and also in pretibial skin cells in the front of the lower leg. For some reason, these T cells fail to recognize the cells in these areas as belonging to 'self' and attack them as if they were foreign. The interaction between the activated T cells and skin cells called fibroblasts causes the release of chemical messengers, called cytokines, into the surrounding tissue. This, in turn, triggers the release of certain proteins, known as heat-shock proteins, the job of which it is to cause cells to multiply and protect themselves from stress. As a result of this cascade of events, the connective tissue within the orbits and in the pretibial skin becomes inflamed, causing the symptoms outlined above.

Carter and Utiger suggest that the close links between hyperthyroidism, Graves' ophthalmopathy and pretibial dermopathy could indicate that, in sufferers, the cells of the thyroid, the orbits and the pretibial skin are coded in such a way that the T-lymphocytes perceive them as being foreign.

Even if this theory is correct, the condition remains puzzling and many questions have yet to be answered. Why, for example, does ophthalmopathy sometimes occur without thyroid disease? Why does Graves' disease often occur without any obvious eye or pretibial involvement? And why is the immune reaction confined to the orbit and the pretibial skin and not affect other parts of the body? The researchers admit to being baffled: no specific gene has yet been found that appears to make sufferers susceptible to the condition. Practically the only clue is that several studies have shown that smoking is a factor.

Getting a Diagnosis

As with so many thyroid problems, it can be difficult to get a diagnosis at first as symptoms can be mistaken for hayfever, conjunctivitis and other eye problems (see Figure 5.5). Graves' sufferer,

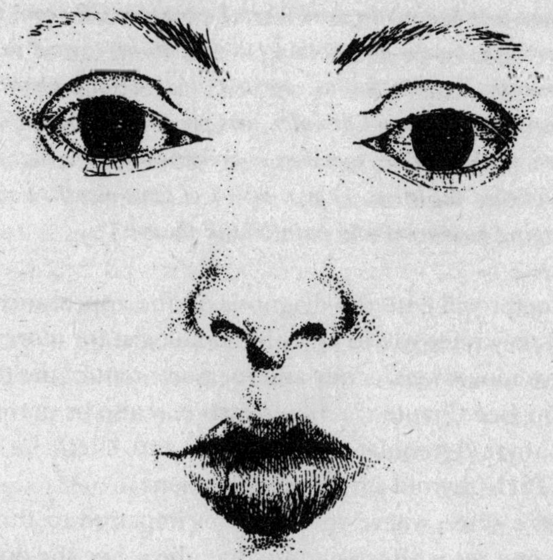

Figure 5.5 *Congestive ophthalmopathy, which is increased pressure caused by swelling, may affect the optic nerves and threaten vision. If you notice this, you should see the doctor immediately.*

Janis Hickey, chair of the British Thyroid Foundation, writing in the association's newsletter recalls:

> *I remember waking up one morning . . . and noticed that my eyes looked and felt peculiar. One GP thought it was conjunctivitis, and prescribed eye drops. When I returned a few weeks later, as there had been no improvement, the GP's response was that conjunctivitis took some time to clear up. I had very bad double vision by the time advice was sought of another GP.*

After the birth of her first baby, Janis had another bout of eye problems:

My vision was bad again, and when I quizzed a GP about this he said, wrongly, that it had nothing to do with my thyroid disorder. Consequently, I went for an eye test and, despite alerting the optometrist to the thyroid disorder, was prescribed a pair of glasses that were of little use; my eyes were so prominent by now that my eyelashes touched the lenses. Over a period of some months I suffered from raging headaches and pain behind the eyes . . . .

The doctor will base the diagnosis on the appearance of your eyes, and may refer you to an ophthalmologist for more detailed tests of eye movement, acuity and measurement of the degree of protrusion (see Chapter 7). Blood tests may also be performed to look for thyroid-stimulating antibodies and check for lowered levels of TSH (thyroid stimulating hormone).

In severe cases, where your vision is impaired or threatened, or where one eye is affected more than the other, the doctor may refer you for more detailed scans, which can confirm a diagnosis and rule out other more serious causes of the symptoms, such as certain types of cancer. The tests can also help the doctor to decide whether medical or surgical treatment is required. The following types of scan may be performed:

- CT (computed tomography) scan *X-rays are taken at different angles and the scanner uses a computer to construct images of 'slices' of the orbit within the skull; the resulting image is clearer than a conventional X-ray picture*

- ultrasound scan *sound waves are bounced off the tissues involved to build up a picture of the size of the tissues and the amount of disease activity*

- MRI (magnetic resonance imaging) *this involves exposing you to short bursts of powerful magnetic fields together with radio waves, which stimulate the tissues to emit radio waves, and these are picked up and analysed by computer to create a 'slice' of the body (because the procedure doesn't involve X-rays it's safer than conventional X-ray and can be performed several times if necessary).*

Disease Activity Score

Some doctors use a special scoring chart, which involves looking for signs of disease activity, such as pain, redness of the eyelids, swollen eyelids and other classic features of inflammation. A score of 3 or more suggests that the inflammatory process is still active.

Helping Yourself

No one likes to receive bad news, but hard though this is, it's as well to prepare yourself for a long, slow haul before your eyes settle down. Left alone, the inflammation does usually gradually subside of its own accord without any special treatment. As your overactive thyroid is treated, any lid retraction, staring and puffiness should gradually ease off. However, as the inflammation dies down and the tissues heal, fibrous scar tissue can form, resulting in permanent problems that can only be treated by cosmetic surgery. Unfortunately, too, eye conditions can often come and go regardless of your thyroid hormone levels. All too often, doctors try to soften the blow by being vague about how long it can take for thyroid eye problems to be resolved, but, as Lucy points out, this may be misplaced kindness:

> *I do wish my consultant had told me how long it would take. I didn't realize how long it would be so I kept hoping. I desperately wanted them to be better for my wedding and when it became obvious that they wouldn't be, I felt bitterly upset and disappointed. I feel more honesty on his behalf would have made it easier to cope with.*

The good news is that there are several things you can do to help yourself.

- Artificial tears or 'comfort' drops, available from optometrists and pharmacies, help moisten the eyes and make them more comfortable.
- Sleeping with the head of your bed raised (put some books under the legs) or propping yourself up on several pillows helps drain away excess fluid and reduce puffiness and swelling around the eyes.
- Diuretics (water tablets) to increase your output of urine may help, too.
- Give up smoking. If you find it difficult, think about joining a stopping smoking support group. Some doctors hold such groups in their surgeries or you could contact one of the private organizations offering stopping smoking courses.
- Mild cases of double vision can be helped by wearing special spectacles with prism lenses. These fit inside your glasses and correct the double vision, allowing you to drive safely.
- Cooling eye masks and gels can help increase comfort.
- Some sufferers find watching TV is easier if they wear a patch over one eye.
- If your appearance worries you, wearing tinted spectacles helps boost your ego by disguising any protrusion.
- Take care with your make-up and grooming. You will feel better if you look good. If your eyes can tolerate it, using a dark eyeshadow, which makes them recede somewhat, can help. Otherwise, try bright lipstick and scarves or necklaces to draw attention away from the eye area.

Incidentally, if you do suffer from double vision or any other eyesight changes, you should let the driving licensing authority know.

Lucy, 32, has found several ways to help herself:

I use a blue gel eye mask which you stick in the fridge which is really soothing. I also wear dark glasses, which cuts the glare of the fluorescent lights at work and also makes me feel less self-conscious. People have got used to me wearing them and I feel much better. I don't use much make-up as a rule, but when I got married, I went to a make-up artist who did wonderful things with my eyes. She used a dark eyeshadow, which she shaded to a darker brown towards the outside and then used bright green on the corners. It looked really effective.

Medical Treatment

In more severe cases, the doctor may decide to treat you with glucocorticoids (often known simply as steroids), which are drugs based on hormones produced by the adrenal glands, and act on the body's fluid balance, hence suppressing swelling and inflammation. As a result, the pain, discomfort, watering and photophobia usually ease too, usually within several days of beginning treatment. Your eyes may bulge less and your vision may improve, though double vision is not usually altered.

The problem with steroids is that the symptoms tend to get worse when you stop taking them or cut down the dose. Some doctors recommend starting such therapy by having two large injections of a steroid called prednisone. Others have found that combining prednisone with other more powerful anti-immune agents is effective.

Sometimes paralysing the restricting muscles by injecting botulinum – a food poisoning toxin that paralyses the nerves that control them (that is, in the muscles) – helps stabilize the eyes and corrects double vision.

Other treatments that may sometimes be recommended include radiotherapy, which can reduce swelling, but doesn't usually relieve protrusion or double vision. However, as this can sometimes cause damage to the retina, it's very much a second-line treatment, used for sufferers who don't respond to drugs, have intolerable side-effects as a result of taking them or who relapse after the dose is reduced.

Finally, cosmetic surgery can be performed to relieve swelling and other symptoms and improve the appearance of the eyes. Such surgery is best kept until the inflammation has died down. The most common type of operation is decompression, an operation to relieve tissue pressure in the orbits by enlarging them so as to allow the swollen tissue to expand. There are various ways of getting to the orbits and the operations are highly specialized. They may involve removing the floor of the orbits from inside the mouth, so as to avoid visible scarring. Such operations are usually carried out by a specialist in orbital surgery, together with a maxillofacial surgeon, ENT or neurosurgical colleague.

One type of operation involves lengthening the muscles that control the lid to correct diplopia. Another operation is called tarsorrhapy, in which the upper and lower eyelids are sewn together, narrowing the opening between the lids, so the eyes look more normal. This also helps to protect the cornea from the damage and infections that can be caused by exposure to the elements. It has to be said that such operations aren't always successful and some sufferers must learn to live with continuing eye problems.

The Best Treatment?

Because so little is known about the disease, there's still quite a degree of disagreement among doctors as to the most effective treatment, but most doctors now agree that the earlier use of steroids and radiotherapy can help prevent more severe cases of thyroid eye disease.

Another controversy revolves around the best treatment for the overactivity of Graves' disease in sufferers whose eyes are affected by the disease. It's been argued that radioactive iodine treatment and surgery could actually aggravate eye symptoms by causing the release antigens (substances the body perceives to be foreign) into the bloodstream. On the other hand, other experts claim that knocking out the thyroid in these ways could improve eye symptoms in the long term by removing some of the antigen. It's also been suggested that antithyroid drugs could be protective during the active phase of eye disease, either because the drugs suppress the immune system or because, by staunching thyroid activity, they reduce the intensity of the immune reaction.

Future Directions

Although the range of options for treating thyroid eye disease is somewhat limited at present, with greater understanding of the processes involved, there's every hope that it will be better treated in the future. Discovery of the precise mechanism involved opens the possibility of using agents that act directly on the immune system. In their review of Graves' ophthalmopathy in the *New England Journal of Medicine,* US Drs Rebecca S. Bahn and Armin E. Heufelder envisage the possibility of using monoclonal antibodies – magic bullets specifically targeted at the cells involved – that would interrupt the cycle of disease at an early stage.

Chapter 6

Baby It's You: Pregnancy, Childbirth and Thyroid Disease

In ancient times, neck enlargement was recognized as a sign of pregnancy. Today, it's known that the thyroid gland plays a major part in the changes of metabolism that go hand in hand with pregnancy. Given the fact that thyroid problems are so common in young women, it's hardly surprising that they often first show up during pregnancy or after childbirth. At the same time, thyroid tests and treatment may be complicated by the normal changes that occur in the thyroid gland during pregnancy.

The changes that take place in your body during pregnancy can improve or worsen existing thyroid disease. Pregnancy can be a factor in sparking off some cases of Graves' disease. In addition, temporary or permanent problems in thyroid functioning often develop after birth and, in particular, a condition called post-partum thyroiditis, or PPT.

Thyroid problems during pregnancy and after birth

- Autoimmune hyperthyroidism – Graves' disease
- Autoimmune hypothyroidism – Hashimoto's disease
- Underactive thyroid after thyroid surgery
- After childbirth – post-partum thyroid disease (PPT): overactivity of the thyroid – PPT, post-partum thyrotoxicosis underactivity of the thyroid – hypothyroidism

The Thyroid During Pregnancy

During pregnancy your whole metabolism changes to enable you to cope with the extra demands placed on your body by the growing baby. The thyroid is crucially involved in this. In the first place the body's production of thyroid hormones goes up. When you first become pregnant, a hormone known as human chorionic gonadotrophin (hCG) produced by the pituitary gland stimulates an increase in the free-floating types of thyroid hormones in the bloodstream. The levels of these fall again towards the end of pregnancy. At the same time, increased levels of the female sex hormone, oestrogen, which is important in many of the changes of pregnancy, causes a doubling of the carrier proteins that transport thyroid hormones around your bloodstream. The body increases the amount of iodine it takes from your diet and the rate at which the kidneys clear iodine from the body speeds up, too. And, at the same time, the level of cholesterol in your blood rises as cholesterol levels are linked both to oestrogen production and to the activity of the thyroid. These hormones are capable of crossing the placenta and are thought to be important in enabling the baby's brain to develop and mature. Certainly a low level of T_4 in early pregnancy is known to damage the development of the baby's brain and lead to cretinism.

This extra burden of work causes your thyroid gland to enlarge slightly – a fact that led to one of the earliest types of pregnancy test. The ancient Egyptians used to tie a reed round the neck of a young woman when she got married and when it broke it was a sign that she was pregnant! Today, the use of hi-tech ultrasound has shown that the thyroid increases in volume by 30 per cent between 18 and 36 weeks of pregnancy.

Your Baby's Thyroid Gland Before Birth

The unborn baby's thyroid gland starts to manufacture its own hormones after 10 to 12 weeks in the womb. Before this, the baby's needs are supplied from your body via the baby's lifeline, the placenta. It's also thought that the baby may be able to absorb thyroid hormones from the liquid in which he or she floats, the amniotic fluid. Levels of the T_4 type of thyroid hormone are low until halfway through pregnancy and steadily rise as pregnancy goes on, while levels of the active T_3 form of hormone are high around mid pregnancy and fall towards birth. Some experts believe this is linked in some way with the maturation of the baby's brain and nervous system.

Stay Warm, Baby

After the baby is born, levels of thyroid stimulating hormone (TSH) produced by his or her pituitary rise abruptly as the baby starts its own independent life, falling to normal levels within a few days afterwards. Babies born at term have a good padding of fat under their skin to help them keep warm. In the first few weeks after birth, the rate at which T_4 is converted into the active T_3 form of thyroid hormone within this fatty tissue, it is suggested, is a crucial factor in the newborn baby's temperature control mechanism.

Hypothyroidism in Pregnancy

Hypothyroid problems are relatively rare during pregnancy, simply because they can lead to difficulty in conceiving.

The most common type of underactive thyroid problem in pregnancy is the autoimmune condition Hashimoto's disease. Alternatively, you may suffer hypothyroidism because you have had thyroid surgery as treatment for an overactive thyroid. The good news is that sufferers from any autoimmune disease – including Hashimoto's – often find that their condition improves during pregnancy. This is because the activity of the immune system dampens down during pregnancy to allow the mother's body to accept the baby, though there's usually a relapse once the baby has been born.

It has to be said, however, that in the past, when thyroid problems weren't so well managed, there was a higher risk of stillbirth, miscarriage, and complications such as pre-eclampsia (the high blood pressure condition associated with pregnancy), bleeding, low birth weight and malformation in babies born to women with hypothyroidism. Today, with the better management of both thyroid problems and complications in pregnancy, there's every chance that you will give birth to a perfectly healthy baby.

Getting a Diagnosis

Diagnosis of an underactive thyroid during pregnancy can be tricky, as even in a straightforward pregnancy, women can experience similar symptoms to hypothyroidism, such as extra sensitivity to cold, coarse hair, difficulties in concentration and irritability. If the doctor suspects that you do have a thyroid problem or if there is a family history of thyroid disease, he or she will probably suggest a blood test to measure levels of TSH, and to check for the presence of tell-tale antibodies.

Treating Hypothyroid Problems During Pregnancy

Whether you already suffer from hypothyroidism when you become pregnant or develop it during pregnancy, you will be prescribed replacement T_4, and the doctor will want to keep a careful eye on you antenatally and during the birth to ensure that you and your baby remain fit and well.

Hyperthyroidism in Pregnancy

Even though thyroid overactivity is more common than underactivity during pregnancy, only about 2 in every 1000 mothers-to-be suffer from the problem. The most common condition is Graves' disease and, again, as with other autoimmune problems, it often improves in late pregnancy only to relapse again after the baby has been born. Overactive (thyrotoxic) nodular goitres – which, as we saw previously, tend to affect older women more often than younger ones – are, as you would expect, a far less common cause of overactivity during pregnancy.

Morning Sickness

One sign of an overactive thyroid may be severe morning sickness – the vomiting and nausea of early pregnancy. Very occasionally, women with an overactive thyroid fall victim to a rare condition known as hyperemesis gravidarum, which causes severe vomiting during the first three months of pregnancy. This is thought to be due to the thyroid-stimulating effect of the early pregnancy hormone, hCG, during the first few weeks of pregnancy. Diagnosis can be complicated by the fact that nausea and vomiting are so common during the early weeks of pregnancy anyway, and also by the fact that hyperthyroidism itself can cause vomiting.

If you do develop severe vomiting (you have difficulty keeping anything down), you should contact the doctor, as you may need to be admitted to hospital. The experts are still debating whether or not women with hyperemesis should be treated with antithyroid pills. Fortunately, hyperemesis gravidarum is rare – only about 5 out of every 1000 pregnant women suffer from it – and, although potentially serious because of the loss of nutrients and the consequent danger of delivering a low birth weight baby, the good news is that it usually clears up during the second three months of pregnancy and always after the baby has been born.

Diagnostic Matters

As with hypothyroidism, it can be difficult to diagnose overactivity of the thyroid during pregnancy as many of the signs and symptoms, such as heat intolerance, rapid heartbeat, nervousness and an enlarged thyroid, occur during normal pregnancy. The doctor will be on the look-out for clues such as eye problems, but a definite diagnosis can only be reached by performing a blood test to determine how well your thyroid is working. If the test also detects thyroid antibodies, it can be a sign that the baby may also develop a temporarily overactive thyroid after birth. This in turn can be a sign that you will be more likely to have thyroid problems after delivery – post-partum thyroid disease.

The Effects on Pregnancy

If an overactive thyroid is untreated during pregnancy, it has to be said that there is a higher risk of miscarriage, low birth weight, stillbirth, and malformation. However, where the problem is picked up in time and treated with antithyroid drugs, you are no more likely than any other mother-to-be to have such problems.

The doctor will choose your treatment carefully to bring the overactivity under control. He or she will want to keep doses of antithyroid pills at the lowest possible level necessary to maintain normal thyroid function. Getting the dosage right is vital as antithyroid drugs cross the placenta and if the amounts taken are too large, this can cause the unborn baby to develop a goitre, which may cause problems during labour and delivery as it may impede the baby's journey down the birth canal or cause breathing difficulties after birth. A large goitre will be able to be seen on an ultrasound scan and, where necessary, a Caesarean section may be planned.

Approximately 1 in 100 babies exposed to antithyroid drugs while they are in the womb develop temporary underactivity of the thyroid gland after birth, a condition known as transient neonatal hypothyroidism (see pages 90 and 92). However, there's no evidence that this adversely affects intellectual development in any way at all.

The doctor will want to monitor your progress carefully and may stop antithyroid drugs during the second three months of your pregnancy. As Graves' disease often clears up of its own accord during pregnancy, it's possible that you may need no further treatment until after the baby is born. If, however, the hyperthyroidism is very severe and doesn't respond to treatment or if treatment creates severe side-effects, it may be suggested that you have thyroid surgery during the second three months of pregnancy. This will definitely be a last resort as there is a slight but definite risk of miscarriage associated with any operation during pregnancy.

Thyroid Disease Developing After Birth

During pregnancy, the action of your immune system is dampened down somewhat in order to prevent your body rejecting the baby as a 'foreign body'. As a result, autoimmune thyroid diseases, such as Graves' disease and Hashimoto's disease, tend to improve late in pregnancy only to get worse again once the baby has been born and your immune system has returned to normal. A very small number – around 3 to 5 per cent – of postnatal thyroid problems are caused by a nodular goitre and inflammation of the thyroid. In another 10 to 15 per cent of cases, problems are due to Graves' disease.

Post-partum Thyroiditis

By far the most common problem after pregnancy is temporary disturbance of thyroid activity known as post-partum thyroiditis (PPT), which is similar to Hashimoto's disease.

The condition was first reported in the *British Medical Journal* by a GP from New Zealand as long ago as 1948, but little attention was paid to it until a study of six Japanese women was published in 1976. This was followed by further research from Japan, Canada, Sweden, the US and, more recently, south Wales and today the condition is a well-recognized syndrome.

No one knows exactly how many women fall victim to PPT – figures of from 2 to 16 in every 100 have been quoted – but the most recent studies suggest between 5 and 9 out of every 100 women run the risk of developing it after having a baby.

What Are the Symptoms?

Typically, the condition strikes around two or three months after the baby's birth and takes the form of an episode of thyroid overactivity. This is followed by a spell of thyroid underactivity, which comes on around four to eight months after the birth. This, too, usually goes away and things return to normal. Some women, however, only experience the overactive phase, while others go straight on to develop symptoms of underactivity.

Although the condition usually resolves itself of its own accord, the syndrome is important because, as endocrinologists Drs John Lazarus and Sakinah Othman of the Department of Medicine, University of Wales College of Medicine, point out in a review in *Clinical Endocrinology* in 1991, as many as 4 out of 10 women who become hypothyroid after giving birth go on to develop permanent thyroid failure by the end of the baby's first year. Another 2 out of 10 women go on to become hypothyroid three or four years later.

A Difficult Diagnosis

Despite its frequency, PPT all too often goes unrecognized because the symptoms of fatigue, lack of energy, dry hair, hair loss, dry skin, difficulty remembering and concentrating and depression are often muddled with the physical and mental changes so many women experience after birth.

Sarah, a 37-year-old social worker, describes how she developed the symptoms of an overactive thyroid after the birth of her second child:

> *I suspect that my problems actually started when I was expecting my baby. I put on hardly any weight during pregnancy and that disappeared as soon as I had the baby. By the time I had my six week check-up, I was feeling very unwell and really not myself. I experienced terrible mood swings. Normally I'm quite jolly and even-tempered, but I was anxious and short-tempered. I would snap people's heads off for the slightest reason. I was constantly rowing with my husband, which again is not like me at all. At other times I would get depressed. I was always tired. And I became very thin, around 6 stone 8 pounds. I suffered from backache. As time went*

on, my muscles became weaker and weaker. If I knelt on the floor, I had to have someone help me back up again. I got terrible palpitations, and I was really worried that I was going to have a heart attack. In the end, it was actually a reflexologist who suggested that I should have my thyroid checked: she could feel enormous crystals in the part of my foot that relates to the thyroid. When I went to the doctor, he diagnosed an overactive thyroid.

Another sufferer, Maggie, 34, who developed an underactive thyroid after her first baby was born, was told by her doctor some months after being diagnosed that she had been suffering from postnatal depression.

Although he's an excellent doctor, I felt he didn't really take my physical complaints seriously. At the hospital, it was clear they thought I was stark raving mad, and I was beginning to feel I was as well.

If you don't feel your doctor is taking you seriously, it's worth persevering and, perhaps, asking for a second opinion. The illness, in its overactive phase, can be confused with Graves' disease. However, unlike Graves' disease, PPT goes away on its own and often no treatment is needed at all, although treatment such as beta-blockers may be useful to control rapid heartbeat. However, if the doctor prescribes antithyroid pills on the assumption that it is Graves' disease, this can be ineffective in PPT and may even speed up the development of the underactive phase.

Graves' disease, of course, needs proper treatment with antithyroid drugs. In the hypothyroid phase, the doctor may prescribe thyroid replacement therapy with T_4 and taper off the dosage gradually over the next few months as the activity of your thyroid returns to normal.

Keeping an Eye on You

The good news is that PPT usually disappears of its own accord given time. The bad is that there is a risk of it reappearing again after future births, so the doctor will want to keep a careful eye on you if you have had it before. The fact that you have suffered PPT should appear on your medical notes, but just in case it gets overlooked, if you do become pregnant again, you should mention it to your doctor and the hospital on your first booking-in visit so that you can get any treatment you may need as early as possible and the midwife and consultant are aware of it.

A Miscarriage Link?

Although PPT normally happens *after* birth, Dr Alex Stagnaro-Green, of the Division of Enocrinology and Metabolism at the Mount Sinai School of Medicine in New York, has recently described the case of a 32-year-old patient who developed a temporary thyroid upset after having a miscarriage following a test-tube baby procedure, IVF – the first time this had been observed. She subsequently went on to give birth to a healthy baby, after which she developed PPT.

In a report published in *Obstetrics and Gynaecology* in 1992, Dr Stagnaro-Green reflects:

> *The lack of research probably reflects a general assumption that gestation must progress to term for the immune changes of pregnancy to be sufficient to allow the expression of thyroid dysfunction in the post-pregnancy period. The present case indicated that the immune changes of the first trimester of pregnancy are sufficient to result in post-miscarriage thyroid dysfunction.*

It's an intriguing study, especially as some other research suggests that recurrent miscarriage and infertility themselves may be linked to the autoimmune process. At the same time, if thyroid upsets occur during the first three months of pregnancy, it raises the fascinating question of whether or not depression following abortion and miscarriage could be linked to thyroid disorder.

Why Does It Happen?

As with so many other thyroid problems, the experts still don't know exactly what causes PPT. However, the presence of thyroid autoantibodies in the blood of sufferers adds to an increasing amount of evidence pointing to a link with the changes that take place in the immune system during pregnancy and after birth. The fact that other autoimmune illnesses, such as rheumatoid arthritis and myasthenia gravis, tend to get better during pregnancy and then rebound with renewed vigour after birth lends weight to this suggestion.

The Depression Connection

Postnatal depression strikes one in ten, though some experts believe the figures are higher, with as many as one in five women being affected, in the year after birth.

In the past, many reasons have been put forward to explain how it comes to develop. These include social and psychological factors, such as relationship difficulties, housing problems, and a previous history of emotional upsets. The latest research, however, suggests that there may be a real physical cause in some cases of postnatal depression: thyroid problems.

A team of doctors led by Dr John Lazarus, of the University of Wales College of Medicine, discovered that women with positive thyroid antibodies have a higher risk of developing mild to moderate depression after birth than women without such antibodies. The team is now looking further into why this should be, as well as trying to prevent the onset of such depression.

Getting Help

Unfortunately, it may be hard to get the help you need with either postnatal depression or PPT, because the rather vague, non-specific symptoms are all too often regarded as being 'normal' in the first few months after birth. Yet, as Table 6.1 (taken from an article that appeared in *Clinical Obstetrics and Gynaecology*) by US doctors Thomas W. Lowe and F. Gary Cunningham, shows women with PPT are far more likely to develop problems such as depression, poor memory and concentration after birth.

***Table 6.1** Incidence of symptoms in women with PPT compared to women with no thyroid problem*

Symptom	%	Phase	% women without thyroid problems
Fatigue	55	Overactive	30 (3 months after birth)
Palpitations	20	Overactive	5 (3 months after birth)
Carelessness/ making mistakes	71	Underactive	11 (3 to 5 months after birth)
Memory loss	71	Underactive	17 (3 to 5 months after birth)
Poor concentration	71	Underactive	6 (3 to 5 months after birth)
Depression	53	Underactive	0 (3 to 5 months after birth)

Dealing with Depression

At a time when everyone expects you to be brimming with happiness, suffering postnatal depression can be a cruel blow. In more serious cases, it may sometimes help to take a short course of antidepressant drugs to correct chemical imbalances in the brain that underlie the depression. However, in milder cases, counselling may be more appropriate. There are also many ways you can help yourself:

- allow yourself to cry or get really angry – calm sometimes follows the storm
- get physical – do some exercise, such as walking, running, dancing, swimming or aerobics
- visit a friend – make it someone who cheers you up
- go out – don't sit at home moping
- visualize your body, imagining energy flowing through it and flowing outwards to your baby and those you love
- keep a selection of songs on hand that you find cheering or uplifting and play them or sing them on those occasions when you need a lift
- if the depression persists, see your doctor, a counsellor or therapist, as drugs or psychotherapy may help

Can I Still Breastfeed?

In the past, mothers taking antithyroid drugs were advised not to breastfeed because of the danger of drugs being passed on to the baby in the breastmilk. Although high concentrations of thyroid drugs have been detected in breastmilk, more recent research suggests that small amounts of the antithyroid drug carbimazole (not more than 30 mg a day), have no effect on the baby's thyroid gland, and that propylthiouracial (PTU) is only found in small quantities in breastmilk. A recent study, reported by Drs John Lazarus and Sakinah Othman, suggests that breastfeeding is safe for babies whose mothers are taking PTU during and after pregnancy. However, methimazole, used to treat hyperthyroidism in North America, is *not* recommended for breastfeeding mothers.

Thus, experts now advise that provided you are only taking low doses of carbimazole, and are aware of the potential risks to your baby, then you may still breastfeed. However, if you plan to breastfeed for very long, your baby's thyroid levels should be regularly checked.

All forms of iodine pass into the breastmilk and can cause the baby to develop a goitre. In the past, women who needed to take radioactive iodine to diagnose thyroid disease have been advised that they can start breastfeeding again after between 1 and 12 days. However, recent reevaluations suggest that it isn't safe to start breastfeeding again before 46 to 56 days afterwards. A newer form of scanning can be used, which allows you to start breastfeeding again after 24 hours, so experts now recommend that this form of scan should be performed if you want to continue feeding your baby yourself.

Antenatal Detection?

Around one in ten women have thyroid autoantibodies in their bloodstream early in pregnancy or shortly after birth. Detecting these autoantibodies could enable doctors to pick out those women at risk of PPT and of postnatal depression so that they could be monitored and treated as soon as possible if they develop problems. Some experts, such as John Lazarus of the University of Wales College of Medicine, have called for the introduction of a simple blood test to screen for thyroid autoantibodies at around 12 weeks of pregnancy. Those with a positive blood test could then be checked for PPT as well as postnatal depression at regular intervals after the birth of their babies. Such screening would enable the mothers to be treated and monitored and prevent the babies succumbing to any potentially negative effects on their mental development.

Other experts, however, argue that, as thyroid problems often don't cause any obvious symptoms (subclinical) and need no treatment, such screening would cause unnecessary anxiety and, in these days of increasing cost-consciousness in the health service, lead to unwarranted extra expense. They claim (though this is arguable) that as women with depression are likely to see the doctor anyway, such screening is not needed.

The jury is still out, but certainly a greater awareness of PPT on the part of doctors would improve the quality of life for women and prevent much unnecessary misery during a time of physical and emotional upheaval.

The Baby in the Womb

You and your baby are so closely interlinked during pregnancy that if you are a thyroid sufferer, substances from your bloodstream, such as antibodies and drugs, can cross the placenta and affect your baby. If you suffer from Graves' disease, for example, autoimmune antibodies, which turn on thyroid activity, may cause your unborn baby to develop an overactive thyroid. Alternatively, if you suffer from Hashimoto's disease, blocking antibodies, which switch off the thyroid gland, may cross the placenta, causing your baby to develop an underactive thyroid.

It may be hard for the doctor to pick up thyroid problems in your unborn baby, but if you have thyroid disease and your baby develops an unduly rapid or slow heartbeat, this can be a clue. Where the doctor suspects there may be a problem, it is possible to measure levels of thyroid hormones in samples of the amniotic fluid the baby floats in by performing an amniocentesis (withdrawing a small amount of the amniotic fluid via a long syringe).

Treatment can be tricky, but if the unborn baby's thyroid is overactive, you may be prescribed antithyroid drugs, which cross the placenta and treat your baby. If you aren't hyperthyroid yourself, you will also be prescribed thyroid hormone replacement, to prevent your own thyroid from becoming underactive.

It is more difficult to treat an underactive thyroid in the unborn baby as only small amounts of thyroid hormones are able to cross the placenta. For this reason, the doctor may prescribe a drug that mimics the activity of thyroid hormone, which is able to cross the placenta more easily.

The Baby After Birth

Much more is known today about the effects the mother's thyroid problems may have on the baby both before and after birth (see Table 6.2) than in the past. If you suffer from Graves' or Hashimoto's disease or have done so in the past, your newborn baby is at risk of developing a temporarily overactive thyroid (transient neonatal hyperthyroidism) because of autoantibodies crossing the placenta. The good news is that as these antibodies pass out of your baby's system during the first three months after birth, the baby's thyroid activity becomes normal.

Neonatal Thyrotoxicosis (Overactive Thyroid)

The baby may seem perfectly well at birth, but develop signs of an overactive thyroid a few days after delivery, once any antithyroid drugs you have taken have passed out of the baby's system.

Some babies have a goitre and the typical protruding eyes of thyroid sufferers. Others may be quite unwell with a rapid heartbeat, be irritable and difficult to settle, develop jaundice, have feeding problems and be slow to put on weight. Tragically, if left untreated, the condition can sometimes prove fatal.

A blood test to evaluate thyroid function and the presence of thyroid-stimulating antibodies can confirm a diagnosis, and the baby can be treated with antithyroid drugs and iodine-containing drugs, together with beta-blockers to regulate the heartbeat. It's still not known for certain whether a brief episode of thyrotoxicosis in a newborn baby has any long-term effects on behaviour or development.

Table 6.2 Thyroid disease and your baby

Baby's problem	Mother's problem	Cause
Fetal hyperthyroidism	Graves' disease	Autoimmune antibodies passing through the placenta
Fetal hypothyroidism	Hashimoto's disease	Autoimmune antibodies crossing the placenta, excess antithyroid pills, or drugs containing iodine
Fetal goitre	Goitre in mother or Hashimoto's disease	Iodine-containing drugs, antithyroid pills, autoimmune antibodies
Neonatal hyperthyroidism	Graves' disease or Hashimoto's disease	Autoimmune antibodies crossing the placenta
Neonatal hypothyroidism	Endemic goitre	Severe iodine shortage, thyroid growth-stimulating antibodies crossing the placenta
	Hashimoto's disease	Autoimmune antibodies crossing the placenta
Neonatal pseudo-hypothyroidism	Drugs taken by mother	Iodine-containing or antithyroid drugs; high thyroid stimulating hormone caused by thyroid stimulating hormone antibodies in the bloodstream

If your baby has a goitre at birth, this may be because your have a goitre yourself and have taken drugs containing iodine or antithyroid pills during pregnancy. Alternatively, it may be due to autoimmune antibodies (produced as a result of Hashimoto's disease) crossing the placenta.

Neonatal Hypothyroidism

The baby's thyroid gland may be underactive at birth, a condition known as neonatal hypothyroidism. This, too, is a result of autoimmune antibodies (which block the activity of the thyroid) crossing the placenta. The condition resolves itself as the antibodies pass out of your baby's system in the first few months after birth. Such transient (passing) neonatal hypothyroidism can also occur in areas of the world where there is not enough iodine in the soil.

More seriously, the baby may be born with an underactive thyroid regardless of any thyroid problem you have. A baby who is short of thyroid hormones for this reason – known as congenital hypothyroidism – and left untreated, will be mentally and physically retarded (cretinism).

Such a problem is usually due to the complete absence of a thyroid gland or failure of the thyroid gland to develop or function properly. This can occur as a result of a faulty immune system, inborn errors of thyroid function, faults in the way the body processes iodine or environmental factors, such as the mother taking certain drugs containing iodine.

Just 1 in every 4000 babies are born with congenital hypothyroidism and treatment with thyroid hormone enables the baby to develop completely normally. Fortunately, too, cretinism has virtually disappeared in developed countries because babies are given a routine blood test five to seven days after birth to measure thyroid function.

In many cases, babies suffering from congenital hypothyroidism appear perfectly normal at delivery. However, in other cases, they may look as if they have spent too long in the womb, the abdomen may be swollen and they may have dry skin. They may also have difficulties keeping warm and develop a dangerously low body temperature (hypothermia) and jaundice. They may have feeding and breathing difficulties, too. A blood test, together with an ultrasound scan to check whether or not the baby has a thyroid, will be performed to confirm a diagnosis, and, if the baby is found to have no thyroid, will be given thyroid replacement therapy immediately, which brings about complete recovery.

Chapter 7

GETTING A DIAGNOSIS

One of the most frustrating experiences, thyroid sufferers find, is quite simply the difficulty of getting a diagnosis. Sufferers with an underactive thyroid often have particular problems, as many classic symptoms of an underactive thyroid, such as depression, weight gain, tiredness and so on are easily attributable to 'stress', getting older, or an inability to cope with life.

It's well-established that women are more likely than men to visit the doctor with often rather vague complaints, which are frequently labelled as depression or 'tired all the time' syndrome. It's also been proved that when women complain of physical symptoms, doctors are more likely to view them as neurotic than they would a man describing the same symptoms. Although the largely male medical establishment has become more sympathetic to women's illnesses in recent years, countless sufferers still describe how their complaints have been met with indifference or been put down to postnatal depression, the menopause and other 'women's problems' at various life stages, such as during adolescence, after childbirth, and the onset of the change of life. It has to be said that, though there are exceptions, all too often doctors give such complaints low priority.

'What Can You Expect at Your Time of Life?'

One sufferer, Angela, 31, relates how, as a teenager, her doctor said her symptoms were due to overeating and, later, another put her symptoms down to a failure to cope with the demands of motherhood:

> *I was overweight from the age of 7 or 8 and I was always on and off diets. Just before my seventeenth birthday, my weight shot up to 11 stone (I'm 5 foot 4 inches) and, despite dieting, it wouldn't shift. My parents were so worried they took me to the doctor. I saw the letter he wrote to the consultant. It read, 'This girl eats too much'.*
>
> *When they did tests, they found I was hypothyroid. I was on thyroxine for years, but then they just took me off it without any explanation and discharged me. My weight continued to yo-yo, but I was fine until I after I had my second baby and the pounds really piled on. Despite the fact that I kept having diarrhoea and I was breast-feeding, I got fatter and fatter. Although at the time I could only see my problem in terms of weight, looking back there were other symptoms of an underactive thyroid: my skin was like elephant hide and if I looked at the wall it looked as if someone was pushing it out at me. It was very disturbing. I was so tired, too, and my short-term memory went to pot. I kept picking up the phone to call someone and then not be able to remember who I'd dialled. When I went to the doctor, he put it down to the fact that I wasn't coping with two children. I remember his words, 'Most tiredness is socio-economic'. It was only when I looked in a medical dictionary and realized that my symptoms fitted those of hypothyroidism that I went back and demanded a thyroid test.*

British endocrinologist Dr Paul Belchetz, writing in the newsletter of the British Thyroid Foundation observes:

Many of the features are non-specific and all too easily lain at the feet of the ageing process itself. They include loss of energy, poor memory, poor concentration and weakness. A whole spectrum of features affects the muscles, joints and nerves and can be thought to be 'rheumatics'. Excessive cold intolerance should alert people to wondering whether thyroid underactivity is present. Each winter the cold weather endangers some elderly people and those with untreated hypothyroidism are known to be especially vulnerable.

Nonetheless, many doctors don't pick up the symptoms of an underactive thyroid.

'I Couldn't Sit Still'

Hyperthyroid problems are easier to diagnose than hypothyroid ones, perhaps because the sufferer is so obviously edgy and hyperactive. However, again, the diagnosis may occasionally be missed if you are older. This is because there may not be the more obvious changes, including eye signs, that are present in younger sufferers. What is more, blood tests aren't always so accurate. Fortunately, Judith's doctor was alert to her symptoms of an overactive thyroid, even though Judith put them down to the start of the menopause:

I was feeling hot all the time, shaky and faint. I thought they were hot flushes and that I was going through the menopause. I was quite shocked when the doctor said I had a classic case of overactive thyroid.

Another sufferer, Donna, writing in the newsletter of the British Thyroid Foundation, relates her experience:

> *I had quite severe hyperthyroidism intermittently for a very long time. I was labelled with 'personality disorder' and prescribed endless Valium for ten years. After the birth of my last baby in 1990, we moved house and my illness came to a head. I went to my new GP with dreadful fear and anxiety symptoms and had lost nearly 3 stone in weight in as many months. He sent me home and very promptly sent a psychiatrist to me who took about ten minutes to make a diagnosis that was later confirmed by blood tests.*

If at First You Don't Succeed

The lesson is that whatever your symptoms are, you must be prepared to persevere. Many doctors are the first to admit that the symptoms of thyroid disease can be confusing. If you start having hot flushes in your forties or fifties, as Judith did, it is perfectly reasonable to suspect that it is the start of the menopause. Similarly, if you feel tired, weepy and emotional after having a baby or a miscarriage, it's not surprising if you or your doctor attribute the problem to postnatal depression.

But whatever the cause of your problems, you do deserve to be listened to. Sadly, some women have to battle for a long time before their doctors take them seriously. This can be difficult enough when you are feeling fit and well, but if you are feeling ill it can be a torment. If you feel you are having problems making yourself heard, you may feel more confident taking a relative or friend with you. Call the surgery to check that the doctor has no objection beforehand.

Talking to the Doctor

Every consultation is a two-way matter. It includes taking a medical history, what you tell the doctor (your symptoms), what the doctor observes (the signs of your condition), a physical examination, tests if necessary, a diagnosis, and advice or treatment.

Before you visit the doctor, decide exactly what you want out of the consultation. It can be quite difficult to remember all your symptoms in an alien environment, when you are anxious or if you are hypothyroid, when confusion and forgetfulness are part of your condition. You may find it helpful to keep a diary and make a note of your symptoms to remind yourself when you visit the surgery, and to write down a list of questions you want to ask the doctor during the consultation. The following list is useful for remembering what to tell the doctor:

- What you have been feeling (your symptoms).
- How this is affecting your daily life.
- What you think may be wrong with you.
- Any fears that you have.
- What you want the doctor to do.
- Any questions you have.
- How you have tried to cope with the problem so far.

You could even tape the entire consultation, though be sure to check that your doctor has no objection beforehand. Some doctors feel inhibited by this, but research has shown that it leads to more careful diagnosis and advice, and also forms a useful record for you to refer back to if you forget anything.

Your Symptoms

First of all, tell the doctor what has been happening to you and how it is affecting your life. Everything you tell the doctor helps to build up a picture that helps with the diagnosis, so be sure not to leave out any symptom, however unconnected it seems to other symptoms. You may think that depilation is a trivial matter more appropriate to the beauty therapist than the doctor's surgery, but if you have noticed that you don't need to remove underarm hair so often, this could well be a clue to an underactive thyroid. Be specific. 'I feel cold all the time' is too vague. Telling the doctor in the height of summer, 'I have to keep the central heating on and switch on the electric blanket before I go to bed', will help make it clear that something is wrong.

It may take just one such symptom to alert the doctor to the possible cause of your condition. In Jennifer's case it was forgetfulness:

> *I'd been going to the doctor constantly with one thing and another. I kept getting sore throats, headaches, and felt tired and weepy, but I was always sent away and being told that it was a virus. I felt that they felt I was just being neurotic. One day, I got so desperate that I wrote everything down and I went in and said, 'I don't want you to say anything, I just want you to listen. My symptoms may seem trivial but I've been experiencing them for a long time now.' The funny thing was that when I mentioned loss of memory, the doctor immediately suggested a thyroid test.*

If you suspect you have a thyroid problem, don't be afraid to suggest to your doctor that this is what you suspect may be behind your problems. You can also ask for the doctor to perform a blood test to check levels of thyroid hormones. Again, what you say may sometimes be the trigger your doctor needs to make a vital connection.

Endocrinologist Dr Paul Belchetz, writing in *British Thyroid Foundation News*, observes:

> *A person should be especially vigilant if there has been any kind of thyroid problem in the past or other members of the family have*

thyroid or some related diseases, such as diabetes, vitiligo, pernicious anaemia.

Alison, 31, recalls that it was mention of her family history that led to her being tested for a thyroid problem:

My mother had had an underactive thyroid and I recognized the symptoms, so when I went to the doctor and asked for a blood test, he was happy to oblige.

There's often the feeling that the doctor's job is to diagnose and the patient's is simply to describe symptoms, but such an approach helps neither you nor the doctor. Effective treatment depends on an open dialogue between you and your doctor. The days of paternalistic doctors are thankfully long gone, and these days most practitioners are aware of the benefits of doctor–patient cooperation. If you feel you can't talk openly and honestly to your doctor, then this suggests that there is a communication problem and you may need to consider seeing another doctor.

The following checklist will help you remember what you want to say once you get to the surgery.

- Your medical history *Include previous illnesses, any history of previous thyroid problems, any family history of thyroid problems, a previous personal or family history of other autoimmune diseases, such as diabetes or pernicious anaemia, as these can sometimes point in the direction of thyroid disease.*

- Your lifestyle *Include details of where you have lived in the past (the soil in some areas lacks iodine and people who have lived in them are more prone to iodine deficiency), your work, your usual personality (thyroid problems often lead to quite dramatic changes in character, so if you are normally vigorous and active and have become slow and sluggish, the doctor needs to know). Tell the doctor what job you do, and what it involves. Thyroid problems can often affect work performance. For example one woman, who is a teacher, recalled how she always missed a particular class because she was so tired.*

- Your eating habits *If you are still piling on weight despite dieting, or if you can't get enough to eat yet are rake thin, this can help the doctor reach a diagnosis.*

- Any other information *If you are trying for a baby, think you may be pregnant or have just had a baby and the doctor doesn't know, you should say so. Tell the doctor, too, about any treatment you are receiving or medicines you are taking. Include over-the-counter drugs and the Pill, as these can sometimes affect the results of blood tests or interact with drugs the doctor may prescribe.*

The Doctor's Observations

Once you have described your symptoms, your doctor will want to ask you some questions to try and build an even fuller picture of your illness. At the same time, the doctor should be paying particular attention to your physical appearance – your weight, the condition of your skin and hair, whether or not your thyroid is enlarged, the appearance of your eyes, even the way you talk and conduct yourself. A hoarse, croaky voice can be a sign of an underactive thyroid, while an anxious, rapid manner can be a sign of overactivity.

Next, the doctor should perform a physical examination to confirm any observations made so far. The doctor will feel your neck carefully, to check whether or not your thyroid gland is enlarged, and may measure its circumference, to check for goitre, take your pulse (a rapid pulse is suggestive of an overactive thyroid, a sluggish one of an underactive one) and your blood pressure. If your eyes are affected, the doctor may use a special measure called an exophthalmometer to ascertain how far they are protruding.

What Happens Next?

If the doctor does suspect that you have thyroid problems, further tests will be arranged to determine the levels of the various hormones put out by the pituitary and the thyroid and to try and find out the exact nature of your problem. The most basic test is a blood test, which is used to measure your hormone levels and this can be performed there and then at the surgery. A single blood test may be sufficient for the doctor to diagnose your problem. However, sometimes you may have to be referred to the hospital for other more sophisticated tests.

Thyroid Function Tests

These tests have changed enormously in the past few years. However, there is still a lot of variation between different laboratories. Three measurements are usually made, of the levels of:

- thyroxine (T_4)
- triiodothyronine (T_3)
- thyroid stimulating hormone (TSH)

This latter hormone, you may remember, is what triggers the thyroid to produce its own hormones. A high level of TSH is suggestive of an underactive thyroid as the pituitary tries to kick-start the struggling thyroid into action. A low level can suggest overactivity, but this measure isn't quite as reliable because pregnancy, pituitary failure and other illnesses that don't involve the thyroid may also result in low levels of this hormone.

The levels of these hormones are then compared to the normal 'reference range', that is, the levels found in a slice of the normal population.

These days it's more common to test the fraction of thyroxine not bound to the proteins that carry it around the bloodstream – so-called 'free thyroxine' – either as a first-line test or if the total thyroxine level is abnormal. Free thyroxine is almost always raised in hyperthyroidism and reduced in hypothyroidism. However, doctors are still arguing as to the best method of measuring free T_4, and the validity of results with some methods of testing.

It has to be said that there is no one, perfect test as thyroid hormone levels are subject to many different influences. For example, factors such as pregnancy, the Pill and other drugs can affect their output.

Measurement of TSH is the most sensitive test for primary hypothyroidism as it starts to rise before T_4 falls below the lower limit. Likewise, highly sensitive TSH tests are able to detect suppression of TSH before thyroid hormone levels are markedly raised in hyperthyroidism.

Different doctors favour different tests, but, essentially, what they are all looking for is the balance between the various hormones produced by the pituitary and/or the thyroid. TSH and the thyroid hormones are like a see-saw – when one is raised, the other is lowered and vice versa. So, for example, if your thyroid is overactive, your T_3 level will be higher, your T_4 level may be higher and your TSH level will be lowered. By contrast, if your thyroid has failed due to underactivity, T_4 is low, T_3 may be low, and TSH will be high. The doctor will use the various measurements, together with your description of how you are feeling, to come to a diagnosis and devise the most appropriate treatment for you.

Reference ranges	T_4 50–160 nmol/l	T_3 1.0–2.9 nmol/l	TSH 0.5–5.5 mU/l
Primary hypothyroidism	↓	↓	↑
Hyperthyroidism	↑	↑	↓

Note: The quoted ranges are for the purposes of illustration, as the exact figures uses vary slightly from laboratory to laboratory

For both hypo- and hyperthyroidism, the TSH is a highly sensitive test of how well your thyroid is working. In some cases, it may be abnormal even though you have no symptoms. In rare cases when the pituitary rather than the thyroid lies at the root of your problems, the TSH may be normal or change in the opposite direction to that shown by the arrows.

Autoantibody Tests

Another blood test may be performed to check for the presence of antibodies against the thyroid. This is done when there is a suspicion of autoimmune problems, such as Hashimoto's and Graves' diseases. Other antibodies known as thyroid-stimulating antibodies, which boost thyroid activity, are present in nine out of ten Graves' disease sufferers and some of those in the early stage of Hashimoto's.

Radioactive Iodine

In the past, before such accurate blood tests were available, doctors often performed a test known as a radioactive iodine uptake test, in which an irradiated form of iodine was given by mouth or injection and the level of radioactivity measured using a special counter to check the amount absorbed by the thyroid gland. As iodine is an essential part of thyroxine, a more rapid uptake than normal could indicate overactivity, as the gland struggled to manufacture thyroxine, while a less rapid than normal uptake is suggestive of underactivity. With the existence of modern blood tests, such tests are performed less often.

Scanning for Problems

The doctor may also want to refer you for various types of scan, to determine the size, shape and texture of your thyroid.

- Ultrasound *Many women are familiar with this from pregnancy. High-frequency sound waves are bounced off the gland to build up a picture on a small screen of the size, shape and texture of the gland. A gel is rubbed on to your neck to make it easier for the sound waves to pass through, and a transducer (an instrument that converts sound waves into electrical signals) is passed over your neck. It takes just a few seconds.*

- Radioisotope scan *This is a special type of X-ray that shows the structure of the thyroid and how it is working. This type of scan is particularly useful for sufferers who have a lump in the thyroid, to check whether it is cancerous or has some other cause.*

- Other scanning methods *Other types of scans, such as magnetic resonance imaging (MRI) and computed tomography (CT), may be performed, especially if you have eye problems (see Chapter 5). Occasionally a conventional X-ray may be performed. Alternatively, if the doctor suspects that the problem originates in the pituitary, you may be given a brain scan.*

Examining the Cells

Another test that can help diagnosis is fine needle aspiration, which is when the doctor removes a few cells from the thyroid gland to examine them under a microscope. The cells are withdrawn using a fine syringe and it is a virtually painless procedure that takes just a few seconds. It has virtually replaced conventional biopsy, in which a small piece of tissue is cut out for examination.

Advice and Treatment

Once the doctor has made a diagnosis, he or she is in a position to suggest the most appropriate treatment and to give you advice on how to manage your condition. The initial therapy is likely to be drug treatment. If you are prescribed medication, it's important to take it exactly as the doctor tells you and to get as much information as possible so that the pills can have the chance to work.

The next chapter deals in more detail with the various types of treatment that are likely to be prescribed for thyroid problems, but before we look at these, there are various questions you should ask.

- *About the type of medication*
  What is the medication for and how is it intended to help me?
  How will I know when it begins to work?

- *About the importance of the medication*
  How important is it to take the tablets?
  What will happen if I don't take them? (Levels of thyroxine build up gradually in the blood, so it may take a while before you feel any effects. Similarly, if you miss the odd dose it probably won't hurt, but if you go on doing so your symptoms will return.)

- *About side-effects*
  Are there any side-effects?

Can I drive after taking them?
Can I take other medicines with them?
Can I drink while taking them?

- *About the future*
  How long do I need to take the tablets?
  When will I need to see you again?
  What will you want to know when I see you?

It often takes considerable trial and error before the doctor manages to find the correct dose for an individual sufferer, so you should be asked to go back for regular check-ups, especially at first.

All medications dispensed nowadays contain a patient information leaflet and this lists the effects of the drug and any potential side-effects. Though these leaflets can occasionally make frightening reading, bear in mind that they have to include all possible side-effects, so many, though listed for the sake of completeness, occur exceedingly rarely. The pharmacist is also a fund of advice on the effects of different drugs. The good news is that, on the whole, the drugs used for the treatment of thyroid problems have a long record of safety.

Giving Advice

As well as offering a diagnosis and prescribing treatment, the doctor should also give you advice on how to cope with your condition. It has to be said that, with the best will in the world, doctors don't always have time and so sometimes information simply doesn't get across.

Research shows that most of us forget what we are told by our doctor. In fact, in one British study, patients had forgotten half of what they had been told within five minutes of leaving the surgery. It's hardly surprising. You are almost certainly anxious and worried about your condition and, at the same time, you are having to deal with the diagnosis of an illness you may only have been, at best, vaguely aware of before.

In the case of thyroid problems there is the added complication that they can fog the brain.

It can help to have things written down, and some practices provide patient leaflets or information booklets for this purpose. If there are no leaflets, write down any advice the doctor gives you in a small notebook that you can refer to, and if anything is not clear, ask the doctor to repeat it or to explain again. You should also ask the doctor if there are any local branches of the various thyroid self-help organizations in your area (see page 176 for the addresses of their head offices). They can offer vital support and also provide information to help you understand your condition.

If You Aren't Satisfied

If you've been trailing backwards and forwards to the doctor for months without being given any helpful advice, or if you feel that you have been fobbed off without any satisfactory explanation of your problem, you may want to get a second opinion.

You can do so by simply going to see another doctor in the same practice or you may want to request to be referred to a specialist. Although some doctors may view such a request as a criticism of their competence, if you approach the matter tactfully by being honest yet assertive, most doctors will be only too happy to arrange an appointment with another doctor or a specialist.

Even if you are happy with your doctor generally, you may feel that, on this particular matter, he or she has a mental block. Many women with thyroid problems relate how they found they got a more sympathetic ear from a female practitioner. Sarah, 37, who developed Addison's disease (failure of the adrenals, an autoimmune condition that is occasionally linked to thyroid problems) following the development of an overactive thyroid, recalls:

By the time I got diagnosed I was virtually at death's door. I had lost so much weight I could barely stand. I had so little energy I used to lie around on the sofa all day. The slightest exertion made me vomit. If I knelt on the floor, someone had to help me up. I kept going down with flu. Every time I went to the doctor, I was fobbed off. When I later read my notes, I was furious at what I saw, because it was clear that they had got me down as neurotic. I thought I was going mad. Eventually, a friend who is a doctor suggested that I should change my doctor, so I did – to a woman doctor. She could see immediately that there was something wrong. When they eventually tested my adrenals, they had completely packed up.

Going Private

UK readers who aren't happy with the advice they have been given may decide to see a specialist endocrinologist privately. The advantage of seeking private treatment is that the doctor is more likely to spend sufficient time examining you, whereas the average NHS appointment with a GP lasts around five minutes. Under current law, there's no obligation for you to obtain your GP's permission before seeking the help of a specialist.

In the UK, doctors are forbidden to advertise, so it can be difficult to know who to consult. If you are on friendly terms with your doctor, you could ask him or her to recommend a suitable specialist. Alternatively, you could check with one of the thyroid support groups for doctors with a special interest in thyroid problems.

To ensure that you get your money's worth, you should prepare for your visit to the specialist carefully, making a note of specific questions you want to ask, tests you may want performed, and listing all your symptoms as above.

Who's who at the hospital

Who	What they do	When you might see them
Cardiologist	A doctor who specializes in the treatment of problems affecting the heart and blood vessels.	If there is any suspicion of heart involvement in your thyroid problem.
Endocrinologist	A doctor who specializes in the treatment of hormone problems.	If it's suspected you have a thyroid problem, if you have serious thyroid disease or develop complications.
Phlebotomist	Someone who takes a blood sample.	When you have a blood test.
Radiologist	Someone who specializes in the treatment of disease by means of radiation from radioactive substances, X-rays or, increasingly, other types of scan.	If you need an X-ray, a radioactive isotope scan or any other type of scan.

Chapter 8

TREATMENT OPTIONS

Once you've been diagnosed, you'll probably feel an enormous sense of relief and look forward to getting the problem sorted out. The positive side is that, compared with some illnesses, thyroid problems are relatively easily and effectively treated. That said, each woman is an individual and it can take some time for treatment for either an underactive or an overactive thyroid to work. It's as well to be prepared for a certain amount of to-ing and fro-ing to the doctor until the most appropriate treatment regimen for you is settled upon. Try not to expect too much too quickly, otherwise you could be in for a disappointment.

Treatment for an Underactive Thyroid

Treatment in this case tends to be the most straightforward. It consists of thyroid replacement therapy with thyroxine (T_4) or, occasionally, triiodothyronine (T_3), which is manufactured in the lab to mimic natural thyroid hormones. In the past, the hormones used to come from animal sources. However, these weren't pure and so today the preparations used are synthetic.

T_3 is chosen for the few sufferers who are unable to absorb T_4 or for those who can't take tablets, as it can be given by injection. Because it is shorter acting than T_4, it is also used when starting treatment for sufferers with cardiovascular problems. T_4 is so similar to the form of the hormone produced by your own body that side-effects are rare, as are hypersensitive reactions.

A Natural Reaction?

Most sufferers seem to tolerate T_4 very well. However, one sufferer I spoke to, Pamela, 68, was adamant that synthetic T_4 didn't work for her. When she was first diagnosed in 1960, she was put on animal thyroid extract and had the following experience with it: 'Literally instant brain function improvement, the fog cleared and the goitre had gone within two months'. When natural thyroid extract was phased out in favour of the synthetic version, however, she found she had headaches and her old symptoms returned. She now survives on animal thyroid imported from Czechoslovakia and other countries, which still use the natural extract. Most doctors today argue that the synthetic version is just as effective as the animal-derived one and preferable because the purity can be guaranteed and dosage is more certain, and Pamela has had quite a struggle to continue getting her supplies. She perseveres, though, as she insists that only natural thyroid extract from animal sources suits her.

Have Patience

Tablets come in three different strengths: 25, 50 and 100 micrograms (mcg). The doctor will generally want to start you on a low dosage to allow your body to get used to it, particularly if you are over 60. The dose will then be gradually increased until you begin to feel better and blood tests show that you are on the amount needed to maintain normal thyroid function. This process can sometimes take several weeks or months, so you will need to be patient until the right dosage is established.

Getting the Dose Right

The doctor will take particular care to achieve the dose that is right for you as too little and your thyroid will continue to be underactive and too much and you will develop signs of overactivity. In the past, sufferers were often given too high a maintenance dose of T_4. Today the general consensus is that the final dose is likely to be in the range of between 50 and 200 mcg, depending on the degree of thyroid failure.

UK doctor Dr Tim Doornan, Consultant Endocrinologist at the Hope Hospital, Salford, cautions, 'Over-quick initiation of thyroid replacement can do more harm than good'. Care is needed because an underactive thyroid causes raised blood cholesterol levels and if these remain high for any length of time, heart disease may result. Starting replacement at a full dose in such a situation, can, he warns, precipitate angina (chest pain) or even a heart attack. And, because T_4 remains in the body for a long time, it's not easy to 'bail out' by stopping the drug. He adds, 'These are not reasons to deny patients the benefits of treatment, rather to tread carefully when starting it'.

As a rule of thumb, the doctor will take into account how long, about, it took you to become hypothyroid, your age and the likelihood of you having underlying heart disease. If you are young and have become hypothyroid soon after surgery or radioactive iodine treatment for hyperthyroidism, the doctor may decide to try you out on a near-full dose of T_4 (100 mcg a day, adjusted upwards according to results of blood tests). If, at the other extreme, you are older or have had severe, long-standing problems, the doctor may start you on a much lower dose, say 25 mcg a day and increase this by 25 mcg every 2 to 4 weeks until the correct level is reached. If you are severely hypothyroid or have heart disease, the doctor should refer you to hospital, as T_4 speeds up your metabolism, including the heart, so it's best to start gradually. If you experience any chest pain after starting on T_4, contact the doctor immediately.

Generally, sufferers are very pleased with the results once the right dose has been found, but it's important not to expect the tablets to solve all your problems. Clare, 39, says:

> *At first I was delighted because I felt much better straight away. It made me realize how awful I felt before. But then I started to feel bad again. I went for another blood test and they upped my dose. This went on for some time until finally I settled on 150 mcg a day, which seems to suit me fine. My periods, which were always somewhat irregular, are now like clockwork. But the tablets don't solve all your problems. For instance, I expected the weight to roll off, but unfortunately it didn't – I'm still going to Weight Watchers. However, I do feel much better. My energy levels are back to normal and I can go out and do everything I used to do beforehand. I do get some joint pains from time to time and I wonder if that's to do with my thyroid, but then you have to accept that as you get older you're not going to be as sprightly as before.*

The Osteoporosis Connection?

Osteoporosis – brittle bone disease – strikes one in four women over the age of 60. It's caused by lack of calcium in the bones and, some doctors believe, lack of collagen (a protein that plumps up the cells in the bone and the skin) in the connective tissue and the bones. It's the cause of much pain and disability as the bones crush and fracture, leading to 'dowager's hump' (a bent back caused by multiple small crush fractures in the spine), plus bones that break easily.

It's long been known that an overactive thyroid can disturb calcium balance and the ability of the body to build strong bones.

More recently, doctors have discovered that people with an underactive thyroid and those with normal thyroid activity with goitres who are being treated with T_4 are also at risk of developing osteoporosis. Worryingly, one group of researchers found a 9 per cent reduction of calcium in the forearms of sufferers who had been treated with T_4 for over 10 years, and a 4 per cent reduction in those who had been treated for more than 5 years. They studied a group of women with thyroid cancer, which had been treated by removal of the thyroid gland plus radioactive iodine (Terrence Diamond, Liza Nery and Ian Hales, 'A Therapeutic Dilemma', *Journal of Clinical Endocrinology and Metabolism*, Vol. 72, No. 6, 1991). Naturally, such complete cessation of thyroid activity meant they had to take T_4 for life. The doctors discovered that both pre-menopausal and post-menopausal women had thinner bones in their thighs and forearms than would be expected, while sufferers who had undergone the menopause also had thinner bones in their spines as well as their forearms. The researchers also measured the presence of a chemical called Gla-protein – a sign of bone turnover – in the blood of the women and discovered that much higher levels were present in those who were being treated with T_4 than normal.

In another study carried out by German doctors that was reported in *Clinical Endocrinology*, also of sufferers being treated with T_4 as a result of surgery for thyroid cancer, 'a significant decrease of bone mineral density' was found in over half of the sufferers, especially in women who had passed the menopause. The interesting thing about this study is that the sufferers had apparently normal levels of thyroid hormones and thyroid function. The researchers suggest that careful monitoring is necessary to determine the lowest dose needed to keep the thyroid functioning normally.

There are many factors involved in the development of osteoporosis, not all of which can be gone into here. On a positive note, however, there are some things you can do to help yourself reduce the risks if you are taking T_4:

- stop smoking
- take plenty of weight-bearing exercise, such as running, dancing, walking as this slightly jars the bones and helps them to become stronger
- once you reach the menopause, consider going on hormone replacement therapy, which helps prevent osteoporosis
- ask your doctor to refer you for regular bone scans to check on your bone density

A Magic Slimming Pill?

It doesn't take much imagination to realize that T_4, by boosting the rate at which your body burns up energy, can produce weight loss. And it has to be admitted that some sufferers do misuse their drugs in this way. As one sufferer who wishes to be anonymous admitted, 'I know I shouldn't, but if I put a bit of weight on, then I step up the thyroxine'. Tempting though it may be, increasing the dose in this way unsupervised is *not* recommended. Apart from the potential for creating unpleasant hyperthyroid symptoms, such as a racing heart, there's also the danger of osteoporosis.

Keep Taking the Tablets

You'll usually be instructed to take the tablets in a single daily dose before you have breakfast. Once the right dose for you has been found, you should experience few problems, so long as you continue to take the tablets. Once treatment has been started, you'll be invited to attend for a check-up after six weeks to check your symptoms and have a blood test to ascertain blood levels of thyroid hormones. This will be followed up a month later, when the results are available. This procedure is continued at monthly intervals until your thyroid function is back to normal, judging both by your symptoms and the results of the blood tests.

Occasionally, sufferers don't respond to T_4, the most common reason being that the medication is being taken incorrectly. Rarer causes include poor-quality thyroid hormone preparations, over-compacted tablets or mistakes in diagnosis.

A Trial of Treatment?

As it's often difficult to distinguish mild underactivity from the silent, subclinical form of hypothyroidism, which has no symptoms, some doctors prefer to institute a trial of treatment for a few months. If your condition improves, treatment may be continued, bearing in mind the power of placebo. If there is no change with treatment, then the doctor will take you off it.

Where the underactivity of your thyroid has come about as the result of a pituitary problem, the doctor will first treat the pituitary and then prescribe T_4. Occasionally, if the underactivity of your thyroid is such that it has affected the functioning of your adrenal glands, the doctor may prescribe steroids (hormones produced by the adrenals) until they have recovered.

A Lifelong Treatment

As your thyroid gland has failed, you will have to carry on taking T_4 for the rest of your life, and you shouldn't stop taking the tablets, except on doctor's orders, even if you develop some other illness in the meantime. It may seem obvious to point out that you should continue your treatment, but it's worth stressing as it's been found that one in ten sufferers actually stop. It can be a nuisance, as Jo describes:

> *I do sometimes feel aggravated by it because it's a continuing reminder that I'm ill, even though I feel better. It's sometimes awkward having to explain it to people if you go away for the weekend, for example, or are sharing a room with someone.*

Needless to say, if you *do* stop taking the tablets, all your old symptoms will return, so it's well worth putting up with the minor inconvenience. You'll usually be advised to have yearly blood checks to ensure that the maintenance dose is still correct. Some areas have developed computerized recall systems to ensure that sufferers continue to be followed up at regular intervals.

Babies and Children

Babies and children with hypothyroidism are also treated with T_4. Treatment should begin within two weeks of birth, and there's no reason for your baby having anything other than a perfectly normal IQ.

Because your child is growing, the doctor will want to monitor progress carefully and the dose will need to be altered as your child grows and develops, as shown in Table 8.1.

***Table 8.1** Recommended T_4 doses for babies and children*

Age	Amount of T_4 per day
0–6 months	25–50 mcg
6–12 months	50-75 mcg
1–5 years	75–100 mcg
6–12 years	100–150 mcg
12 years	100–200 mcg

These doses may need to be modified according to the weight of your child.

Treatment for an Overactive Thyroid

Treatment for hyperthyroid problems tends to be more complicated than treatment for an underactive thyroid, and demands more patience from the sufferer. Most sufferers say that their symptoms started to improve within a month or so after treatment began, but it often takes as long as a year or more before they feel completely back to normal.

Many sufferers continue to feel vaguely unwell for some time after tests show that their thyroid has returned to normal. This is because the condition tends to come and go, and response to treatment can be unpredictable and variable. It has to be said that only a third of sufferers who take antithyroid drugs go into remission and, of these, two-thirds subsequently develop further attacks of hyperthyroidism. For this reason, in the UK, you will usually be referred to an endocrinologist or a doctor who specializes specifically in thyroid problems rather than being treated by your GP. Elsewhere, in places such as the US, you are likely to already be under the care of an endocrinologist.

Stages of Treatment

Treatment consists of three stages. First, the doctor will try to bring your symptoms under control, through the use of antithyroid drugs, and, for many sufferers, this is all that is needed to restore the thyroid to normal. Second, the doctor will try to restore your thyroid to normal functioning in an effort to bring about a remission, in other words to free you from recurring symptoms so you can come off the drugs. The problem is that the drugs often don't bring about a permanent cure. If you relapse – and around half of all sufferers treated with antithyroid drugs do – the doctor may talk to you about surgery to remove part or all of your thyroid. The precise choice of treat-

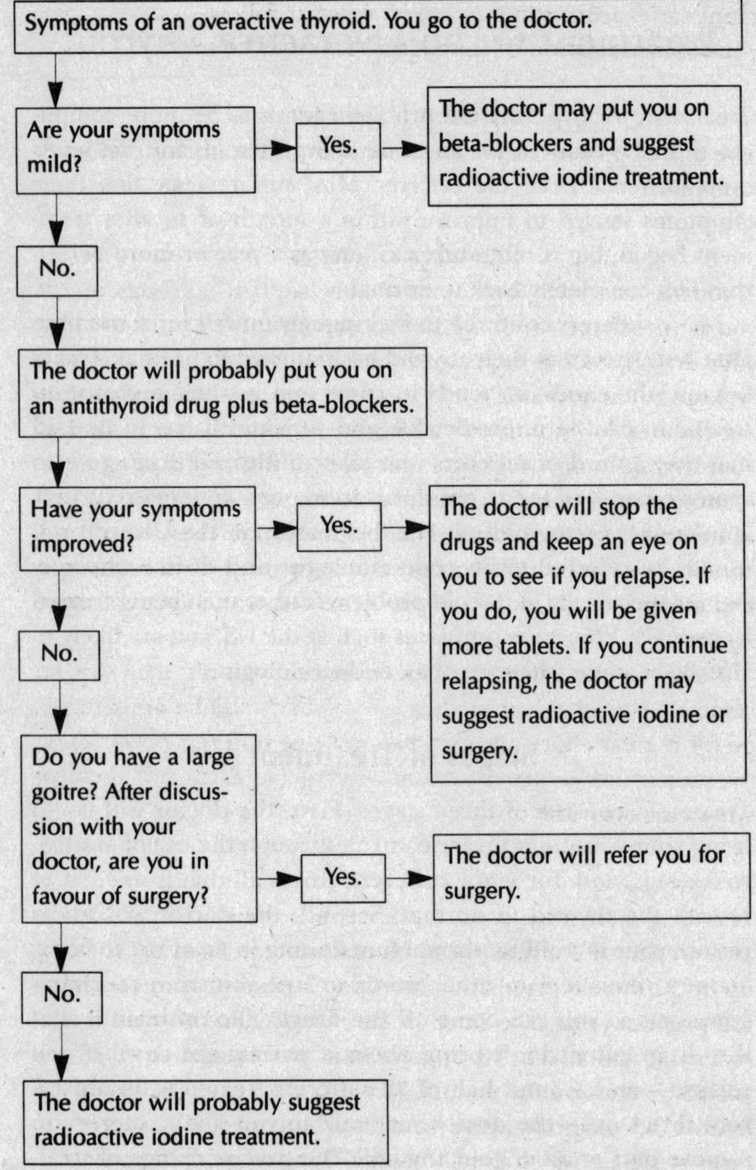
Symptoms of an overactive thyroid. You go to the doctor.
Are your symptoms mild?
Yes.
The doctor may put you on beta-blockers and suggest radioactive iodine treatment.
No.
The doctor will probably put you on an antithyroid drug plus beta-blockers.
Have your symptoms improved?
Yes.
The doctor will stop the drugs and keep an eye on you to see if you relapse. If you do, you will be given more tablets. If you continue relapsing, the doctor may suggest radioactive iodine or surgery.
No.
Do you have a large goitre? After discussion with your doctor, are you in favour of surgery?
Yes.
The doctor will refer you for surgery.
No.
The doctor will probably suggest radioactive iodine treatment.

ment varies from clinic to clinic, so what follows is just to give you some indication of the regime that may be tried.

Sorting It All Out

The chart opposite shows you what options the doctor may want to explore.

Antithyroid Drugs

If you are under 18, the doctor will use antithyroid drugs, and if you are pregnant, drugs are also the treatment of choice to bring your thyroid back to normal as quickly as possible. The dose will be kept as low as possible and treatment stopped altogether during the last few months of pregnancy. If your disease is mild, if your thyroid is only slightly enlarged or if you prefer drug treatment to other types of therapy, the doctor may well suggest a trial of treatment for a year to see how you respond. However, if your condition is not brought under control by antithyroid drugs on a first attempt, it's likely to relapse on subsequent courses of treatment, too.

Being on the drugs can be a nuisance: you must be sure to remember to take your medication regularly and be prepared to go for regular check-ups. As a result, some sufferers prefer to go for radioactive iodine treatment or surgery, which rids them of symptoms once and for all.

Carbimazole

The drug most often used, carbimazole prevents the production or secretion of T_4. It works by blocking iodine from being taken up by the thyroid gland and preventing further steps in the chemical processes that take place in the manufacture of thyroid hormones. It also affects the autoimmune process and so cuts back antibody attack on the thyroid. In the US, the drug used is methimazole (a biologically active form of carbimazole). It's taken in the form of tablets, which usually contain 5 mg of active ingredient.

Block and Replace

The doctor will first prescribe carbimazole and, once your thyroid has been brought back to normal, may then add in a small dose of T_4 in a 'block and replace' regime. This means that the activity of the thyroid is suppressed by the action of the carbimazole and the T_4 is given to prevent development of symptoms of hypothyroidism. Such a regime is said to lead to smoother control of your condition, fewer visits to the surgery once it's established and the avoidance of any tests during the course of treatment. Block and replace is not suitable during pregnancy because of the dangers of exposing the baby to T_4.

Different doctors favour different approaches and some prefer to bring the thyroid rapidly under control, then to gradually taper off the dose over the next four to eight weeks, depending on your response to treatment, until you are on a maintenance dose of 10 to 15 mg a day. However, other doctors believe this method is less reliable, as there are often wide fluctuations in thyroid function.

Possible Side-effects

Although you may take carbimazole with no problems at all, it's as well to be aware that there can be some side-effects. These include nausea, hair loss and skin rashes. If you do, it's worth mentioning them to the doctor as it may be possible to adjust the therapy or put you on a different drug.

In about 1 in 1000 cases, it can lead to a serious condition called agranulocytosis, in which the number of white blood cells, which combat infection, is lowered. The symptoms of this are high temperature, sore throat, mouth ulcers, and, if it is allowed to progress, it can lead to bronchopneumonia. So long as the condition is picked up early and you stop taking the drug, it is reversible. If you develop any of these symptoms while on carbimazole, *you should stop taking the tablets and contact the doctor at once*, who will perform a blood count and put you on antibiotics to kill the infection, until your blood count returns to normal.

Propylthiouracil (PTU)

If such a reaction should occur, an alternative drug called propylthiouracil can be prescribed, which is far less likely to cause agranulocytosis. Like carbimazole it prevents the production or secretion of T_4 by preventing the uptake of iodine by the thyroid gland. It also prevents T_4 from being converted into T_3 in certain tissues. It's taken in tablet form and, again, the doctor will usually start with a high dosage and taper this off until you reach a maintenance dose.

Similar side-effects to carbimazole may occur – there may be nausea and headache, and, occasionally, jaundice or hair loss. An itching rash may be a sign that you need alternative treatment.

The drug should *not* be given to anyone with obstruction of the breathing passages, for example, such as would be caused by a large goitre, and it should only be used with extreme caution during pregnancy, while you are breastfeeding or if you have poor kidney function.

Beta-blockers

These are drugs used to regularize the heartbeat and to relieve the symptoms of anxiety caused by an excess of adrenalin in your bloodstream. If your thyroid is severely overactive, to the extent that you have developed a thyroid crisis – palpitations, sweating or extreme nervousness – the doctor may prescribe beta-blockers as well as antithyroid drugs.

Propranolol

The most commonly used beta-blocker is a drug called propranolol, which works by blocking the effects of adrenalin in the body, so slowing your heartbeat, and it may also limit conversion of T_4 into the active T_3 form of thyroid hormone. It comes in the form of pills, sustained slow-release capsules or can be given by injection. You may be started on treatment to relieve symptoms while the doctor awaits the results of blood tests. The doctor will gradually taper off the treatment as the antithyroid medication starts to work. However, because beta-blockers quell symptoms of overactivity, the doctor will have to rely on blood tests from now on to determine levels of thyroid hormones in your blood.

Side-effects

As well as slowing the heart rate, the drug can cause the air passages to go into spasm, causing wheeziness. This can be serious if you have asthma or heart failure. It can also cause stomach upsets and tingling or numbness of fingers and toes. Others complain of lack of energy, sleep disturbance and bad dreams. It should never be given to you if you have any serious form of heart disease or asthma, and should be prescribed with caution if you are known to have impaired liver or kidney function, towards the end of pregnancy or during breastfeeding.

Who Relapses?

The main trouble with antithyroid drugs is that the thyroid may become overactive again after treatment. This is particularly likely to happen if your gland is very enlarged or you have needed large doses of drugs to bring your overactivity under control. If a relapse is going to happen, it usually does so within a year of coming off treatment, and you can recognize it by a return of some or all of your original symptoms. Sometimes friends or your partner may be the first to notice that you are becoming hyperthyroid again. If you do think you have relapsed, see the doctor, who will arrange for further blood tests and treatment.

Surgical Options

If drug treatment does not succeed in bringing thyroid overactivity under control, if you have a large goitre, particularly if it is pressing on your windpipe, or a medium-sized goitre that bothers you, if you cannot take antithyroid drugs or simply don't wish to or if you are planning to have a baby, the doctor may suggest thyroid surgery to bring your condition under control.

These days, a partial thyroidectomy, in which most of the thyroid is cut out, is considered to be an effective treatment for hyperthyroidism, provided the surgeon is skilled. If you do decide to opt for surgery, it's worth taking some time to ensure that you are operated on by a surgeon who is experienced in performing such operations. Your doctor may be able to suggest someone in your area or will be able to refer you to a hospital that specializes in such problems. Alternatively, you could contact one of the self-help groups for the names of surgeons who are known to specialize in the operation (see page 176 for some addresses).

Is It a Good Idea?

Surgery restores normal thyroid function for most of those who have it. For this reason, many doctors believe that all young women with an overactive thyroid should be offered it, so that they can go on to have a family with no further worries. However, around one in five sufferers who have the operation go on to become hypothyroid – usually in the first 2 years after surgery – and 5 in 100 continue to experience recurrent episodes of overactivity from time to time.

In the past, when surgical techniques were not so well developed, damage to the parathyroid glands deep within the thyroid gland, which are responsible for controlling calcium balance in the body, could occur. There's also an extremely small risk of damaging the nerves that supply the vocal cords. In experienced hands, such complications are rare today.

What Happens

In a partial thyroidectomy, around two-thirds of each of the two lobes of the thyroid are removed. Before the operation, your doctor will want to bring your thyroid levels to normal by means of antithyroid drugs and iodine compounds, such as Lugol's iodine – a solution of iodine and potassium iodide in water. You'll be examined to make sure your vocal cords are normal, and an anaesthetist will also come to check you over before your operation to determine the amount of general anaesthetic that you will need.

In the operating theatre, you are given a general anaesthetic and the doctor makes a curved incision in your neck along one of the creases, so it is less likely to show up after it has healed. The underlying layers of skin and muscle are drawn aside to expose the thyroid. The doctor then carefully detaches the gland from its blood supply and cuts away three-quarters to seven-eighths of the gland, taking care to avoid nearby nerves and seal off blood vessels. Most surgeons prefer to remove more rather than less of the thyroid, to avoid recurring episodes of overactivity and the need for subsequent surgery. Tubes may be placed in the site of the removed gland to drain off any blood that gathers there, and the doctor then replaces the layers of muscle and skin and stitches or clips together the cut.

After the operation, you will need to stay in hospital for a short time – usually from two to five days – and you can expect to feel some soreness. Tubes are inserted into the thyroid for a day or so after the operation to drain off any blood.

After you return home, your progress will be followed up at regular intervals to check on your thyroid function. If you are one of the one in five who develop hypothyroidism as a result of the operation, the doctor will treat you as for hypothyroidism, with thyroid replacement therapy.

The scar usually fades gradually until it looks like a fine line on your neck.

After-effects

Thyroid surgery is usually extremely successful. However, occasionally some sufferers have a type of skin that is prone to producing a lumpy form of scar tissue, which is especially likely if you are of African or West Indian origin. A clue as to whether or not this is likely to happen is if other wounds have healed to form a lumpy scar.

Other sufferers sometimes develop a hoarse voice after the operation, due to bruising of the nerves that supply the vocal cords during surgery, but this usually passes over the next few weeks or months. Some temporary damage to a nerve occurs in around 1 in 50 cases. More rarely – in around 1 in 500 cases – the surgeon may accidentally cut a nerve, which results in permanent hoarseness. If you use your voice in your job, for example if you are a singer or a teacher, you may want to think carefully before opting for surgery as there is a chance that your voice could be less strong and have a tendency to wobble after surgery.

Another rare consequence is damage to the parathyroid glands, which lie hidden deep within the thyroid. If these become bruised during the operation, you may develop a condition called tetany, due to low blood levels of calcium in the blood. The first sign is numbness and tingling around the mouth, followed by muscle weakness and cramp in the hands and feet. Treatment consists of calcium tablets or injections, together with vitamin D. Symptoms usually disappear as parathyroid function settles back to normal. However, if the parathyroids have become damaged, as happens very occasionally, long-term calcium supplementation is necessary.

'I Feel Better Than I Have for Years'

Many sufferers are delighted by the operation and just wonder why they took so long to have it. Angie, 48, an administrator, had suffered with an overactive thyroid for years:

I was really quite ill. On one occasion I had to spend 48 hours in hospital because I kept passing out through having palpitations. The antithyroid drugs just didn't work – as fast as they gave them to me, I went overactive.

Eventually, it was suggested that I had radioactive iodine, but I just didn't like the sound of it, so the doctor suggested a thyroidectomy. I went to see the surgeon on the Friday and I was in hospital having it on the Monday. The operation only took about three-quarters of an hour, I spent a week in hospital and had a week off work and then I went back.

Immediately afterwards my voice got lower, which is apparently quite common, but it's back to normal now. I also noticed alarming bruising all over my chest when I first had a bath after having the operation. Apparently they have to strap you down – but no one told me and it was rather frightening.

I'm absolutely delighted I had it done. It's a beautifully neat job and I feel better than I have for years.

Helping Yourself

Preparing for Surgery

Most conventional doctors don't give advice on getting yourself fit for surgery. However, it stands to reason that if you are as healthy as you can be before going for surgery, you will enhance your chances of a quick recovery.

Try to cut out alcohol and junk foods for a month before you go into hospital, so as to put less of a strain on your liver. It could be a good idea to drink less coffee, tea, cocoa, cola and other drinks high in caffeine for a while, too. It's been found that those who consume a lot of caffeine tend to recover more slowly from anaesthetics.

Eat plenty of fresh fruit and vegetables, which are rich in the vitamins and minerals your body needs to help repair itself. Vitamin C, found in all fresh fruit and vegetables, is particularly good for tissue healing. Raw foods supply instant energy and are also easier for your digestive system to cope with than processed foods. Eat regularly and properly to avoid wild fluctuations in blood sugar levels, which exaggerate ups and downs in how much energy you have.

In Russian hospitals, the herb ginseng is regularly given to patients who are recovering from operations. It is said to have balancing effects on the metabolism, which could make it especially suitable for thyroid sufferers.

It's also worth practising relaxation and avoiding stress before and after your operation, as this too can hinder recovery. Controlled breathing, such as that used in yoga, can help your body get rid of anaesthetic gases more quickly and also help you have a better night's sleep – something that isn't always easy in hospital.

In some hospitals in the US, hypnosis is used for surgical patients. Anaesthetists say that hypnotized patients need less anaesthetic and fewer painkillers after surgery. It can also help you feel more self-confident and recover more quickly.

In his book *How to Survive Medical Treatment*, medical scientist Dr Stephen Fulder suggests that women should opt to be operated on in the middle of the menstrual cycle – from days 7 to 20 – when resistance is highest, and not during a period, when the body tends to be at its lowest ebb.

Finally, pack a bottle of the homoeopathic remedy Arnica in the suitcase you take to hospital. It's superb for any type of trauma and can help ease bruising and discomfort after any operation.

After the Operation

Convalescence is a time for regenerating the body's healing powers and restoring your weakened immune system. Again, a good diet is vital for this work of repair and regeneration.

Foods should be light and nourishing, yet easy on the digestion. To this end, avoid large quantities of red meat, which is difficult to digest, and steer clear of fried or fatty foods for the same reason.

Vitamin C, as already mentioned, is especially good for helping wounds to heal, while the mineral zinc, found in seafood, liver, yeast and seeds, helps boost the immune system and aids tissue repair. The B vitamins can help relieve stress and may prevent nausea and vomiting after surgery.

In their book *Superfoods*, naturopath Michael van Straten and Barbara Griggs suggest the following foods as being particularly nutritious in convalescence:

- Fruits *apples, blackcurrants, dates, grapes, kiwi fruit, lemons, oranges, raspberries*
- Vegetables *carrots, spinach*
- Grains *oats, barley, millet*
- Seeds, nuts *almonds, chestnuts*
- Herbs *garlic*

There are other things you can do to speed up recovery. Wheatgerm oil and vitamin E, massaged over the site of the incision once it has started to heal, can help prevent scarring.

In some hospitals, nurses are using aromatherapy oils to help patients mentally and physically. Neroli and lavender are especially useful to lift stress and ease anxiety. They can be burned in a burner, dripped on to your handkerchief or pillow or dropped into your bath.

Radioactive Iodine Therapy

This consists of a tasteless drink or capsule, which, over the course of weeks or months, calms down the activity of your thyroid. In the past, radioactive iodine therapy was only used for sufferers over 40. However, today doctors are increasingly using it for younger sufferers as it is both convenient and simple. The doctor may suggest it if:

- you have problems taking antithyroid drugs for any reason
- you have relapsed after having drug treatment or thyroid surgery
- you prefer this type of treatment and cannot become pregnant because you have had a hysterectomy or been sterilized
- you undertake not to become pregnant for at least a year after being given therapy
- you are older and your cardiovascular system is under strain from the overactivity of your thyroid, or any other situations in which surgery would be risky

The iodine is taken up by cells in your thyroid and the radioactivity then knocks out the cells that are overactive, bringing your thyroid function back to normal.

This doesn't always work and more courses of radioactive iodine treatment may be needed. For this reason, some doctors prefer to give a dose that will cause your thyroid to become completely inactive. This is because an underactive gland is easier to treat than an overactive one. In this case, the doctor will inform you of this plan and you will have to attend the clinic at monthly intervals, so that your blood levels of thyroid hormones can be monitored to prevent your thyroid becoming severely underactive.

Such a course of action is effective in eight out of ten cases within three months. However, if your thyroid function has not returned to normal or become underactive by four months after treatment, the treatment will be repeated.

Your overactive thyroid will be brought under control by giving you propranolol and carbimazole, to avoid you developing thyroid crisis due to the large number of thyroid hormones that are released into the blood as the thyroid cells are destroyed. The propranolol is continued to control symptoms, but the carbimazole will probably only be stopped a few days before radioactive iodine treatment is given as the gland has to be working at the time of treatment. They will be resumed around seven to ten days afterwards, once the radioactive iodine has cleared from the urine, and continued until the cells are destroyed. This should happen within about six to ten weeks.

Is It Safe?

Given the known links between exposure to radioactivity and cancer, sufferers often wonder whether or not there are any risks attached to radioactive iodine therapy.

The treatment has been used for a long time – over 40 years in some countries – and there is no evidence of any danger of developing cancer or leukaemia. However, only you can decide if it is for you.

The treatment may sometimes cause thyroid crisis, or thyroid storm, due to excessive release of hormones as the cells die off. The treatment is also controversial in that some experts believe that thyroid eye disease can become worse after radioactive iodine therapy. Occasionally, too, sufferers who have been treated with radioactive iodine develop harmless nodules some years after treatment. And sometimes the treatment causes inflammation of the thyroid (thyroiditis). Fortunately, this is usually temporary.

The treatment shouldn't be used if you are pregnant or likely to become pregnant in the near future or if you are breastfeeding, as it can permanently damage your baby's thyroid.

Coping with Treatment

Although radioactive iodine is perfectly safe for sufferers of thyroid overactivity, it can affect the thyroid function of people with normal thyroids. For this reason, you will have to be isolated for a week or so, usually in hospital, until the dose has cleared from your body. If you are being treated with lower doses, however, as often happens during second or subsequent treatments, you may be able to be treated at home, provided you undertake to limit your contact with others. This means not spending more than an hour in a public place or on public transport, keeping your distance from babies or young children and avoiding kissing and other close contact with your partner, friends or relatives, particularly women of childbearing age, until the radioactivity has cleared from your system.

Smaller doses still can be taken over two to four weeks, and without these precautions, so long as your job doesn't involve contact with radioactivity. Even then, try to avoid holding babies or young children for a few days after treatment.

All this can be very stressful, as Maggie, 34, discovered:

> *I found the radioactive iodine treatment especially traumatic. I developed diarrhoea and sickness, nose bleeds, sore gums and my skin looked grey and ashen. But it was the emotions that surfaced that caused me most pain. I was put in isolation, away from the other patients, and I went through every feeling imaginable – depression, anger, the lot. It was horrible not being able to have any contact with anybody. I knew the treatment was necessary, but I had problems with the idea of it. I used to be an active antinuclear campaigner and now here I was drinking the stuff.*
>
> *The second time I had to have radioactive iodine, I spent two weeks in isolation at home. It was totally different. Even though I couldn't sleep in the same room as my partner, I was with my family, I could make phone calls, walk around the garden and feel much more normal.*

Being kind to yourself and giving yourself little treats, like a new book, massaging your own feet or shoulders with aromatherapy oils or watching a good video, can help you to cope. Plan some bigger treats that you can do with others for when you are clear of the radioactivity. For example, a weekend away with your partner or a friend, a short holiday, a professional massage, pedicure or facial.

After Treatment

After treatment, the doctor will want to perform routine checks to ensure that your thyroid function has settled down, and to keep a look-out for signs of hypothyroidism. There's also some evidence that eye problems may be more common in those who have had radioactive iodine treatment.

A common regime is for you to go back to the clinic three or four times in the year after treatment, twice in the second year, and once a year after that.

Treatment for Thyroiditis

In mild cases of viral thyroiditis, no treatment may be necessary. Alternatively, anti-inflammatory drugs, such as aspirin, can help. If you are in prolonged pain, the doctor may prescribe steroids for a month or so, gradually tailing off the dose as you get better.

If your thyroid gland has been damaged as a result of autoimmune thyroiditis, you will be treated for hypothyroidism (see above).

Post-partum Thyroiditis (PPT)

See Chapter 6.

Lumps and Bumps

If you have a goitre, particularly if it is small, soft and causing no symptoms, no treatment is usually necessary. However, if you have developed a single hot nodule, or a multinodular goitre, you may be offered a partial thyroidectomy, or lobectomy, to remove the overactive part of the gland. Alternatively you may be offered radioactive iodine therapy.

Surgery may also be performed if you have a thyroid adenoma, a harmless thyroid tumour. Surgery is also necessary if you have thyroid cancer (the operation will be followed by radioactive iodine treatment, particularly for certain types of thyroid cancer most likely to affect older women, and external radiotherapy).

Thyroid Eye Disease

See Chapter 5.

Treatment chart

Type of treatment	What it does	Used for
Antithyroid drugs	Prevents excess formation of hormones	Overactive thyroid, Graves' disease, PPT
Beta-blockers	Lowers heart rate	Overactive thyroid, PPT
Thyroid replacement therapy	Replaces thyroid hormone	Underactive thyroid, PPT, following thyroid surgery, following radioactive iodine treatment, following autoimmune thyroiditis
Lugol's iodine	Used as an iodine supplement	Severe hyperthyroidism and especially before thyroid surgery
Radioactive iodine therapy	Kills overactive cells	Overactive thyroid, Graves' disease, after thyroid surgery, single hot nodule, thyroid cancer
Surgery	Removes part of thyroid	Overactive thyroid, Graves' disease, thyroid nodules, multinodular goitre, thyroid adenoma, thyroid cancer
Cosmetic surgery	To sew the eyelids together or enlarge the orbits	Thyroid eye problems

Chapter 9

'I Just Want to Feel Normal Again' – Learning to Live with Thyroid Problems

As far as many doctors are concerned, thyroid disease is fairly straightforward – you do some tests, come to a diagnosis, treat the problem, end of story. The picture from the other side of the doctor's desk often looks very different. Although it is often a tremendous relief to know what is wrong with you, a diagnosis is just the beginning. Learning to live with the knowledge that you have a long-term condition can be immensely challenging.

Apart from anything else, discovering you are suffering from a chronic illness is often an enormous blow to the self-confidence. You may come to distrust your body and to feel alienated from it for behaving in such an unpredictable way. The realization that you may have to be on treatment and have regular check-ups for the rest of your life can be hard to cope with, too. You resent your increasing dependency on the medical profession, on others, and the loss of your individual freedom. Although the people caring for you may be trying to be kind, because they are familiar with the disease, and are often rushed, they may be unaware of how you are feeling and the distress you have bottled up inside.

Maggie, 34, who has an overactive thyroid, speaks for many sufferers when she says:

I can't believe it has come from nowhere and it's taken over my life. I'm taking pills every day. I feel totally out of control. I never imagined it would be like this. I just want to be well again. I'm sick of pills and hospital.

Living with Loss

Every time we go through any change in our lives, we experience loss. And with this comes grief. In the case of thyroid disease, there are many losses to deal with. As well as the very real physical suffering, there is the loss of your self-image as a fit, healthy person. One sufferer writes:

My hearing loss is devastating. Conversation is difficult, especially at social gatherings, and I don't go to pubs any more. I still wonder how I manage to hold down a job, considering I can hardly remember who I have just dialled on the telephone, let alone hear them. Getting up in the morning is arduous. I still have skin like elephant hide. My puffy face and hooded eyelids have given my face a grotesque, mask-like quality.

Appearance Matters

These physical effects of thyroid disease can be especially hard to bear in a culture where everyone is judged to some extent by their appearance, and women in particular are valued for their looks. Sufferers with severe eye problems often describe how unattractive they feel, as do those whose hair has become thin. Others have to cope with unacceptable weight gain or loss. In a culture where being fat is particularly frowned upon, even putting on just a little weight can seriously dent the body image, as one sufferer, Angela, describes:

I am painfully aware of society's disapproval of my abundant flesh. I find myself rushing at the earliest opportunity to tell acquaintances that I'm fat because I'm ill, not because I overeat, honest. Some people are sympathetic, but a woman once said I was using my illness 'as an excuse'. I don't eat much at parties in case someone is watching me.

And although losing weight is generally viewed as being more desirable, being 'too thin' can occasionally lead to sufferers being wrongly labelled anorexic. A doctor writing in the *British Medical Journal*, describes the case of Anne, a hypothyroidism sufferer and running champion, whose descent into Addison's disease [an autoimmune illness that, though rare, is known to affect some thyroid problem sufferers] went unrecognized until she was at death's door by friends and medical staff alike:

People said she was a nutcase, that she had invented the running glories and nicked the trophies. Perhaps she had anorexia nervosa. Perhaps, I wondered, her thyrotoxicosis was fictitious. The more we labelled her problem as functional [having no physical cause], the more she fitted the mould. I still have the article clipped from a psychiatric journal that seemed to describe her symptoms and behaviour perfectly.

If you have a large, noticeable goitre or if you have to have surgery, all these things can result in loss of self-confidence, feelings of loss and the accompanying grief. As Peter Speck says in his book *Loss, Grief and Medicine* (Baillière Tindall):

If the body image is disrupted by . . . surgery, it can lead to a grief-like reaction, which requires a period of mourning before the resulting trauma is resolved and a new, acceptable, body image is formed. The acceptance of this by others is important.

At the same time, other medical conditions, such as reproductive problems, that accompany thyroid disease can bring additional difficulties of their own. If you want to have a baby, but have been unable to conceive, you may feel a loss of status and purpose in life. You may feel as though it's your 'fault' if you and your partner had planned a family. If, as some sufferers do, you have a miscarriage or stillbirth, this can result in feelings of failure as a woman. Alternatively, if you have a baby and it has a birth defect or problem with its own thyroid, this can also lead to feelings of grief and guilt.

Emotional Aspects

Thyroid disease in itself can cause you to be moodier than usual and, at the same time, can lead to a loss of mental sharpness and lack of interest in everyday life. Rapid fluctuations in thyroid levels are particularly liable to lead to mood swings. And some treatments used for thyroid problems can have psychological effects. For example, beta-blockers can make you feel slowed down and mentally foggy. Even when you have been treated, it can take some time before you feel yourself again. It's important to give yourself time to accept what has happened to you and not to expect too much of yourself.

All Nicely Under Control?

Unfortunately, sufferers can often see things in a very different way to the way in which their doctors see them, as you will see from Judith's comments. The impact of the disease on sufferers' lives and the uncertainties of treatment can create a heavy emotional toll:

Most of the time I work from home, which is fine, but every so often I have to go to town for a meeting. I get terribly panicky about it, wondering whether I'm going to be OK that day. In one way, being self-employed helps – I can take it easier when I have to – but, on the other hand, if I don't work I don't get paid and that's a real worry. I suspect if I had a regular job I'd have had to have had a lot of time off. My consultant said to me somewhat casually, 'It'll probably end in surgery'. All the time I was thinking, 'How am I going to fit that in?' As soon as they say, 'It's very common among middle-aged women', it's as though it's not serious. The other week I saw a doctor for a check-up who said, 'Oh, it's all nicely under control, isn't it?' I said, 'No, it isn't'.

Doctors who are experienced in treating thyroid problems should be aware of such factors. However, some doctors may not be so aware and may not take you seriously. Either way, you may find that talking about your problems to other sufferers or some form of counselling or therapy is helpful. In some cases, a short course of antidepressants may help. There's no need to feel a failure if you take these. They can often tide you over a rocky period and help you regain your emotional balance. And antidepressants, unlike tranquillizers, are not addictive.

Treatment Trials

Medical diagnosis and treatment is frequently stressful, especially as it can take time to reach an accurate diagnosis and treatment may take time to take effect. A hospital stay, which you may need if you have to have radioactive iodine treatment or surgery, is stressful, too, involving as it does the loss of familiar surroundings, social contacts and autonomy. In Chapter 8, Maggie, 34, vividly described the sense of isolation and confusion she experienced during a five-week stay in hospital, and how having a second round of radioactive iodine treatment at home rather than hospital enabled her to feel happier and more in control. Discussing alternative treatment options with your doctor can be similarly empowering.

Hospitals are institutions – large, complicated and hierarchical. They have to be administered so that the whole machine operates smoothly. In a busy hospital clinic or ward with so much going on, it's easy to feel lost, alone and isolated. Away from your own familiar surroundings and in the grip of an illness that is hard to understand, you naturally feel terrifyingly powerless and depressed. Finding out more about your illness by reading about it or, when you feel up to it, joining a self-help group and getting to know other sufferers can enable you to discuss your treatment in a more informed way with your doctor and enable you to feel less of a victim.

However, some women prefer not to know too much about their illness. They fear that it might depress them. Accept the way you are feeling and do what you feel is right for you.

Feeling Out of Control

Time and again, women suffering from thyroid problems complained that they felt their needs and wishes were ignored or trivialized because they weren't 'textbook' cases. Maggie, 34, recalls:

> *After I took the first tablet, I took my baby to the park. I was sitting in a cafe having a coffee when, suddenly, I experienced a terrible hot flush and a prickling sensation in my body. I felt really peculiar. The sensations came in waves. Then, when I went to bed, I had muscle spasms in my thighs. I felt really panicky. Another time, when I was in the post office, I came over all faint. I was very frightened, wondering how on earth I was going to get home. Eventually I went back to the doctor, who told me it was psychosomatic. He said that it took three months to get a response to thyroxine and that I couldn't possibly be having a response in three hours.*

I was in floods of tears. I could see that he just thought I was being neurotic.

Eventually I got the doctor to agree to give me a blood test before the usual three months (the time the dose normally takes to build up to its optimum level). My thyroid count had gone up almost to normal. They were astonished at how quickly my blood had taken it up. And I felt that vindicated me.

From the medical staff's point of the view, so long as the hormonal measurements are within the expected range, there is no problem. But, as Judith observes, an illness that can lead you to feel perfectly well one day and terrible the next can be particularly undermining, because you never know what to expect. For women who are used to managing their own lives, everything can appear frighteningly out of control, even when, medically, the doctor perceives treatment to be proceeding well.

Personality Counts

Feelings can be a particular problem with any thyroid condition as the illness itself can lead to changes in your usual behaviour and personality. Time and again, sufferers describe behaving and feeling in ways that are uncharacteristic for them. For example, becoming lethargic and depressed when they are normally energetic and lively, arguing with people close to them, when normally they are placid, being unable to think straight. Try to accept that such feelings are a normal part of your condition, and don't expect too much of yourself. You *will* feel better, but, in the meantime, put off any major decisions until your condition is medically under control.

Regaining Your Confidence

It may be a little while before you learn to trust your body again. Accept that it takes time, but rest assured that, as your condition is brought under control and you begin to feel better, you will be able to deal with all the changes it has brought about in your life and healing in a much wider sense begins to take place. Many sufferers find that as they learn to live with their condition, they also learn new ways of thinking about their illness in the context of their lives. The Chinese word for 'crisis' means two things: 'danger' and 'opportunity'. If you can see your illness, however unwelcome, as opening up the prospect of positive growth and development, you will find it much easier to cope.

Psychologists describe several stages in learning to deal with life transitions, such as the development of a chronic illness. At first, there is immobilization: you feel numb, out of control and unable to act. Next, comes minimization, when you may describe your problem as something trivial or deny it altogether. This is followed by a period of self-doubt and depression as the reality sinks in. The low point in self-esteem is acceptance or letting go, when the reality of your new situation really hits home and you begin to realize the limits it may place on the way you lead your life.

However, as with so many changes, once you hit rock bottom, you begin to go up again. Your self-esteem begins to rise as you test your new situation and start to make positive changes in your life. Such changes can be something simple, like joining an exercise class or deciding to eat more healthily. Alternatively, they can be more far-reaching. Jan, for example, decided to train to be a counsellor and did a course in psychology. The new insights she gained helped her make sense of her own problems as well as giving her a potential new career.

At the same time, you begin search for meaning in your condition at a deeper level. Angela, writes:

Being ill has revealed to me a resilience I never knew I had, has taught me to value the good things in my life – my children, my friends. Now I take nothing for granted, no one at face value. I have gained a tiny insight into the even more serious illnesses that befall people and recognize their real courage in adversity. I begin to understand the isolation that can be felt by the differently abled in a torso-obsessed culture.

Another sufferer, who went through a period of depression, says:

I always used to be rather impatient of people who were depressed, and think it was just a matter of them snapping out of it. When I experienced it myself, I realized it wasn't like that. I am now much more tolerant of friends who are depressed.

Such insights help you to 'internalize' the change, make it part of you and move on, a changed but enriched person. Many self-help and voluntary organizations have been started by people who had feelings they needed to deal with and experiences they felt would benefit others.

Dealing with Emotions

The first step in dealing with any emotion is to recognize and acknowledge it. Once you have pinpointed *what* you are feeling, find ways to give vent to it. If you are angry, shout, scream or make animal noises. Hit a cushion, beanbag or mattress, tear up telephone directories, blow up balloons and jump on them. Walk along a beach or by a river and hurl stones into the water, saying what you are angry about with each one. If you are unhappy, cry. Lay in a store of tissues, play some sad music. Really get into your sadness. If you are frightened or anxious, feel these feelings, too. Think about your fears and experience the feelings they bring, let the feeling of fear wash over you in waves, accept it and observe it as it diminishes. Realize that, although it can make you feel bad, it can't destroy you. Experiment with affirmations, positive thoughts that you choose to think instead of negative, undermining ones. Repeat to yourself phrases such as 'I choose love' – the opposite of anger or fear – or find an uplifting poem or passage from a book to copy out and stick up where you can see it. Explore your relationship with your illness. Imagine it as a person and try writing to it and write its replies back to you; or sit it on a cushion and talk to it and imagine it replying to you.

Dealing with Practicalities

Once you have calmed down, do something practical to deal with your feelings and emotions. If you are unhappy with your treatment, write a letter of complaint. If you still don't feel well despite treatment, make an appointment to see the doctor to discuss what further treatment options might be available. Find out as much as you can about your illness, so you can understand what the doctor says to you, and you can be involved in the management of your condition. Keep a written record of physical symptoms and a note of any medical treatment you are on.

Dr Rowan Hillson in her book *Thyroid Disorders* suggests measuring your neck monthly if you have a goitre, monitoring your weight and taking your pulse every so often to check its regularity and whether it is getting faster or slower. She also counsels sufferers to become aware of their physical appearance, and any factors that may be signs of the gland becoming over- or underactive, such as temperature preferences, patterns of tiredness, appetite, bowel motions, periods and so on. She writes:

> *It can be difficult to recall what happened when, and which pills you took for how long. But if you have written notes of things you*

can measure, like your weight and pulse, as well as how you feel, you can see if your thyroid function is speeding up, slowing down or steady.

Such actions, as well as being useful, can help you feel much more in control. It's easy to go on to automatic pilot when receiving medical treatment and not really confront your illness. By consciously monitoring your own condition and participating in your treatment, you will feel much more in control. And once you feel better, reach out and make contact with other people. Joining a support group for people with your condition can help you feel less alienated.

Looking After Yourself

Developing any chronic illness can offer an opportunity to look at your life and the way you live it. All too often, women rush around caring for others and putting their own needs last. They skip meals, miss out on vital sleep and neglect their own physical and emotional needs. It's especially important if you are depressed to look after yourself physically. Get plenty of sleep, but if you don't find it easy to drop off, don't lie there worrying about it. Get up and do some housework, write some letters.

Diet Matters

If you are feeling depressed or tired, it can be hard to eat well. However, a healthy diet can not only help you to feel better physically, it can also be a way of enabling you to feel more in control of your life.

In general, you should eat the sort of diet now recommended for health. This means aiming to get at least five helpings of fruit and vegetables a day, and some experts now say we should aim for nine. At the same time, you should be cutting down on saturated fats and replacing them with monounsaturated and polyunsaturated fats, found in olive oil, nuts, seeds and oily fish. Carbohydrates are burned easily by the body, so fill yourself up with wholemeal bread, rice, pasta, baked potatoes. According to nutritional doctor Stephen Davies, people with an overactive thyroid have increased demands for certain nutrients, especially the B complex of vitamins, which are known to combat stress, and trace minerals. Also, B_{12}, found in liver, beef, pork, eggs, milk, cheese, and kidneys, is particularly important in combatting a form of anaemia called pernicious anaemia, which thyroid sufferers are especially at risk of contracting. B_{12} is also involved in focusing and visual sensitivity, which may be of relevance to sufferers with thyroid eye problems. Focusing depends on the action of your muscles, and image transmission is a process that requires energy.

Calcium – found in dairy foods, soya beans, sardines, salmon, peanuts, walnuts, sunflower seeds, dried beans and green leafy vegetables – is also important to thyroid sufferers, especially in view of the continued debate about the risks of osteoporosis. Calcium is also important for a regular heartbeat, helping metabolize iron and aiding the transmission of nerve impulses. As we have seen, calcitonin, which is involved in regulating calcium levels in the blood, is one of the thyroid hormones. Magnesium – found in figs, lemons, grapefruit, sweetcorn, almonds, nuts, seeds, dark green vegetables and apples – is needed, too, to help metabolize calcium. It's also an aid in fighting depression, and helping promote a healthier cardiovascular system.

Manganese – found in nuts, green leafy vegetables, peas, beetroot, egg yolks, wholegrain cereals – is another vital mineral. It's involved in the formation of thyroxine, and can help eliminate fatigue, aid in muscle reflexes, improve memory and reduce nervous irritability. You can get all these nutrients by paying close attention to your diet. You may also want to consider taking a daily multivitamin/mineral tablet, or a vitamin B complex supplement.

Try not to skip meals, as this can lead to low blood sugar and aggravate feelings of tiredness and lack of energy. If you are lacking in energy and don't feel up to shopping or cooking, enlist the help of your partner or a friend. If you can't find anyone to cook for you, go to the supermarket and stock up on dishes that you can put in your freezer. Treat yourself to a few meals you especially like or get in some pasta and some ready-made sauces for a virtually instant meal. On occasions when you are feeling more energetic, use the time to batch-cook a few favourite dishes and freeze them. With a simple salad and some fruit, you have the makings of a meal.

Smoking and Drinking

If you like a drink, there's no reason for you to avoid alcohol, so long as you stick to safe limits of no more than 14 units a week (a unit is a glass of wine, half a beer or lager or a single measure of spirits).

However, as everyone is aware, smoking is bad for your health. It may be particularly harmful for thyroid sufferers, given the strong connections with thyroid eye disease. The latest research shows that smoking is even more harmful for women than it is for men, and one in two smokers will eventually die of a cigarette-linked disease. Heart disease is a particular risk, given the fact that thyroid sufferers are at increased risk of heart problems and high cholesterol (a risk factor for heart disease) in the first place. All good reasons to kick the weed if you possibly can. The evidence is that if you give up before the age of 35, your risks of dying of smoking-linked illnesses are no greater than for any other non-smoker.

It's all very well for the experts to advise giving up smoking, but not so easy if you are a smoker to actually do it. Women in particular smoke to relieve stress and to avoid weight gain – this last factor being a particular problem if you are hypothyroid. In order to stop smoking, you need to *want* to give up. The health benefits of stopping smoking are clear, especially if you suffer from thyroid problems, while thinking of what you could do with the money you save, and perhaps setting aside the money you spend on cigarettes to treat yourself to a holiday, a course of massage treatment or whatever, may be an added incentive. Giving up with your partner or a friend can help keep up flagging motivation.

You may need special help in identifying why you carry on smoking and finding ways to stop. Some doctors hold clinics for those giving up smoking. Alternatively, you may want to attend one of the many private stop-smoking courses that are now available. Hypnotherapy can also help some smokers.

A Sense of Balance

It's especially important if you are ill to balance the body's need for activity with rest and relaxation. Exercise can help keep your heart, lungs and muscles in good working order. However, thyroid disease can lead to problems exercising. Muscles may be weak due to hyperthyroidism or hypothyroidism. Your joints may ache and you may become easily tired and breathless. Despite such difficulties, everyone can benefit from exercise – it's simply a matter of finding the type that is right for you. Gentle activities, such as walking, swimming or yoga, can be especially invigorating, particularly if you are feeling tired. But any such exercise needs to be tailored to you as an individual, so take expert advice from your doctor before embarking on any exercise programme.

Exercise has additional mental benefits. It releases hormone-like substances in the body called endorphins, which help you to feel calmer and more relaxed. And, by increasing your stamina and the ability of your heart to work harder, an exercise programme can actually give you more energy.

Exercising with a friend can aid motivation, but don't push yourself too hard. Recognize your limits, especially when you first begin to exercise. As you get stronger and feel more energetic, you will be able to take on more. If you are joining a gym or embarking on a formal exercise programme, again, you should consult your doctor beforehand to check whether your chosen activity is suitable, and explain your thyroid problems to the trainer or instructor.

Increasing Well-being

When you are feeling down, it can be hard to feel that anything is going well. Think about how you have dealt with adversity in the past and tell yourself, 'I got through that, I can get through this'.

Every day, make a list of things that have gone well. There's always at least a little something – a chat with a friend, someone who smiled at you, a TV programme you enjoyed. Jan describes an encounter in the pharmacy that gave her renewed hope when she was feeling miserable:

> *I was standing waiting to be served and she came up to me and said, 'I know what's wrong with you. You've got Graves' disease'. She then said, 'I had eyes just like yours'. I looked at her and her eyes were perfect. It was just what I needed to enable me to believe that things would get better.*

Then, think of all the things that have upset you or made you angry and allow yourself to feel those feelings, too. When you've cleared these negative feelings, think of the next thing you are looking forward to – a cup of herbal tea, a book you want to read, a radio programme you want to listen to, something small you plan to buy. Think about your outside environment and how it affects your moods. Don't leave the curtains closed during the day. Put a bright cushion, picture or postcard of somewhere you have been or would like to go where you can see it. Be aware of sounds and the effect they have on you. TV programmes and song lyrics can affect you subconsciously. If you are feeling depressed or down, now is not the time to watch a programme about death or disaster or listen to depressing music (unless you are using it as an aid to enable you to feel blocked emotions, see above). When you are feeling vulnerable, try playing something relaxing or uplifting, such as dance music. Dance around your sitting room if you have the energy, sing or hum along inside your head or even out loud.

Your Relationship

Any change, especially illness, can affect close relationships, such as the one with your partner. Married or not we all have a series of unwritten agreements with our partners. If something happens to disrupt these, for example if it's been assumed that you are very independent, if you are always the one who takes responsibility for taking the children swimming, entertaining the boss, being the bright, cheerful coping partner, and then this changes through tiredness or illness, it can put even the most stable of relationships under serious strain.

Men, in particular, seem to have more problems dealing with illness than women: to experience feelings of weakness or fear can threaten a man's sense of masculinity. They often feel they should be the protectors in a family and experience a sense of failure when something like an illness reveals to them their powerlessness.

Many sufferers described how their relationships came under pressure as a result of personality changes, changes in physical appearance and physical disability, too. Changes in sex drive and activity as well as changes in the number of arguments you have with your partner (both common in thyroid disorders) are among the factors psychologists pinpoint as being particularly stressful in charts devised to quantify the impact of life changes.

- Be gentle with yourself and your partner, and recognize that it takes time to adjust to any new situation.
- Talk to your partner about your condition and the many ways in which it may affect you. However, try not to let it dominate your life once the medical problems have been sorted out. Do things you enjoy together, such as going for a meal, for a walk, to the cinema, on holiday and forget about your illness for a while.
- Be sensitive to your partner's personality style and recognize that the way he will deal with your illness is the same as the way he deals with other difficult situations in his life. Don't expect him to behave in the same way as you.
- If your partner is not sympathetic, find a sympathetic ear among your friends or seek out a counsellor or therapist to help you deal with your feelings.
- Recognize that every relationship has its ups and downs. Don't blow these out of proportion, and try to believe in your ability to pull through. Try to avoid minor irritants becoming major issues. Talk about them and try to be patient.

Treat Yourself Better

The lack of self-esteem that accompanies illness can make it hard to give to yourself. At the same time, if you feel physically unattractive, you may feel you don't want to bother with clothes or make-up. Looking after yourself and pampering yourself in small ways, though, can make a real difference to how you feel, as well as helping you to look better, which, in turn, can make you feel better. If you catch yourself feeling guilty about spending money or time on yourself, tell yourself you are worth it. Even something small like buying a beautiful scarf to hide a goitre or a scar on your neck can do wonders for your self-esteem.

- If your hair is thinning, look after it by going for regular haircuts and washing and conditioning it regularly. Improving your diet and taking exercise can help lessen hair loss, while various hair products, such as mousses, can be used to thicken it and give added volume. The chemical process of colouring can add volume, too, as can a good cut or a root perm, which can create lift and fullness. Thinning hair tends to look fuller if you keep it short.

- Make wearing hats or scarves a part of your personal style. Alternatively, think about investing in a wig. There are some very convincing ones available, so no one need ever know you are wearing one.

- Clever make-up can help you disguise coarse skin and protruding eyes. If your skin is dry, invest in a good moisturizer. A visit to a beauty salon, or at least the cosmetics counter at your local department store, to help you choose the most suitable make-up, can be a worthwhile investment, too.

- Matt eyeshadow looks best on your eyelids, as a high shine draws attention to them. Remember, too, that light colours draw the eye forward, while dark ones push the eyes back. Use concealer to disguise under-eye puffiness, and an eyebrow pencil to apply short, feathery strokes to make sparse eyebrows look thicker.

- Play up your lips to draw attention away from your eyes. Use a lip liner to define the edges. Use a blusher to achieve a delicate, natural glow, lifting a pale or grey-looking complexion.

- Treat yourself to a massage. As well as soothing away stress and tension, allowing someone to touch you can help you accept yourself and make you feel better about your body and the way you look. A facial massage can help disperse excess fluid around the eyes and rid the tissues of toxins. Don't put oil around your eyes, though, as it can burn the skin.

- Go easy on yourself emotionally. Avoid self-messages with the words 'I should', 'I ought' or 'I must'. Instead, be kind to yourself, allowing yourself to make choices with words like 'I could'. Accept that you will never be exactly the same as you were before you developed thyroid problems, but believe that life can still be good.

- Most of us revert to being like children when we are going through emotionally difficult experiences. Pander to your inner child, buy yourself a fluffy toy, or something else to cuddle.

- Make a list of things you like to do, then tick those you have done in the past week. Do something new for yourself each week. Buy yourself a bunch of flowers, wear a new perfume, treat yourself to a walk in the park, a trip to the cinema. Take time out to relax, or try some meditation.

If you've just been diagnosed, it may seem as though you will never feel better. However, all the people I spoke to while writing this book have come to terms with their thyroid problems and now enjoy life – and so can you.

Chapter 10

ALTERNATIVE WAYS WITH THYROID PROBLEMS

A growing number of people have turned to alternative or complementary therapies for help with medical problems. Orthodox medicine deals well with acute problems, that is, those illnesses that can be diagnosed, treated and then go away. The trouble is, as medicine has conquered the great scourges of the past, such as TB, polio and other infectious illnesses, a growing proportion of diseases – and thyroid disease is one of them – are chronic or long-term. This type of illness, though fairly straightforward to treat in some ways, is not so well remedied by orthodox treatment. Effective medical treatment is available, of course, and you may well feel a new woman once the appropriate treatment has been found for your thyroid problems. However, as with all chronic illnesses, thyroid problems can take several months or even years to sort out. In the meantime, at best, your symptoms may be alleviated or prevented from progressing. At worst there may be relapses, side-effects and little or no improvement. The doctor may become tired of hearing your tale of unremitting woe and you may be frustrated that the doctor doesn't appear to listen or take your problems seriously.

Donna Beckwith, writing in *British Thyroid Foundation News*, echoes the feelings of many sufferers when she says:

> *Although looked at in clinical medical terms thyroid disease is basically straightforward and fairly easy to treat, often the reality of the symptoms during times of imbalance are much more difficult to live with and can be very distressing . . . . Knowing your blood levels are OK doesn't help much when you're feeling dreadful.*

The fact is, there is more to physical illness than what can be measured and it's here that alternative or complementary therapies can be a real help. Good healers of every persuasion have always paid attention to more than simply the relief of symptoms. The existence of placebo effects – the phenomenon whereby illnesses improve whatever the treatment – is proof of the power of the mind over the body. What alternative or complementary medicine does is recognize that the influences on health don't stop at the door of the doctor's surgery, and that there are more ways of helping sufferers than treatment with drugs or performing surgery.

A Whole Person

What all the alternative, or complementary, therapies do is to see you as a whole person, not just a set of symptoms. And this outlook is particularly relevant to those with thyroid problems, where the effects of the disease are so wide-ranging. While the average visit to an orthodox doctor takes just ten minutes, most of which is spent scribbling on your notes or writing a prescription, when you visit an alternative or complementary practitioner you are likely to spend a long time talking and discussing things about you that may seem unrelated to your thyroid – details about your work, home life, diet, state of mind, relationships, your ways of spending free time, the ups and downs of your health in the past, and the health of the rest of your family, will all be sought. The aim of this is to give the practitioner a whole picture of you as a person.

Partners in Healing

Another difference between orthodox and alternative medicine is that when you visit a complementary practitioner, you become an active participant in your treatment. When you are treated by an orthodox practitioner, you tend to be a passive recipient – literally a patient – of the treatment meted out to you. The therapies complementary therapists offer, however, demand your involvement. You may be asked to make a change in your diet, your exercise habits or other aspects of your lifestyle. This can be tremendously empowering, especially when you have a condition in which your body sometimes seems to be running you rather than the other way around.

A Matter of Balance

Another feature of most alternative therapies is that they are concerned with balance. It will be clear from reading the rest of this book that thyroid problems are very much about a question of balance. According to any number of non-conventional therapies, illness is seen as being caused by an imbalance and by the body's attempts to right itself. It's not hard to see how such ideas can be applied to thyroid disease.

In herbalism, for example, the ancient concepts of 'hot' and 'cold' characteristics as related to disease fit in perfectly with the insights of twentieth-century endocrinology into thyroid disease. A hot condition is likely to have a high metabolic rate and feel hot, stressed and nervous. Someone with a cold condition, on the other hand, will feel cold, have a sluggish metabolism and a tendency to be overweight.

Acupuncture, too, views all illness as a disturbance in the balance of two opposing qualities – yin and yang (see below). And, although the endocrine system is not recognized as such by Chinese medicine, there are a few studies showing that acupuncture can be successful in treating several hormonally based disorders, particularly infertility due to hormonal imbalances.

Which Therapy?

So, what types of alternative or complementary therapy might be most beneficial?

As thyroid problems have such an impact on the mind as well as the body, therapies that act on the body via the mind, and vice versa, are likely to be particularly helpful. For example, meditation and yoga can help calm overactivity of the brain, which is often a problem for sufferers of hyperthyroidism. Hypnotherapy may also be useful, helping you learn to relax more easily. Therapies such as T'ai chi, sometimes known as moving meditation, and, again, yoga can raise dwindling energy levels, which may be a problem for hypothyroidism sufferers. Massage can help you feel cared for, something that is especially valued when you suffer from a chronic illness. Aromatherapy is likely to be helpful, too, as the essential oils work gently on the mind as well as the body to rebalance energy and mood. Rosemary, for example, is invigorating and helps relax away tension, basil lifts your mood and helps you feel alert, lavender is relaxing, and lemon balm can help you if you have difficulties sleeping.

These are only a few suggestions to start you thinking. When it comes to choosing an alternative therapy, it's very much a matter of experimenting and finding the one that suits you personally. As so many of these therapies work better if you are in a positive frame of mind about them, using a therapy you find appealing is a powerful part of treatment. Below you'll find details of some therapies that may be particularly suited to the treatment of thyroid problems, because their underlying philosophies in some way relate to the idea of balance. However, they are not meant to be in any way prescriptive, so if you like the idea of trying a particular complementary therapy, apply a little trial and error until you find the one that is most helpful to you.

A Matter of Energy

Acupuncture is very much concerned with rebalancing energy levels.

According to Chinese medicine, disease occurs when the body's internal balance is disrupted in some way. Harmony and balance depend on the smooth flow of the body's life force, or energy, known in Chinese medicine as *ch'i.* This circulates along invisible pathways or channels. The smooth flow of energy also depends on the correct balance of two qualities known as yin and yang in the body. Yin, the feminine principle, is associated with coldness, darkness, wetness, softness, while yang is linked with the more masculine qualities of hardness, brightness, heat, dryness. Illness can be due to excessive cold, or yin, in the body, bringing about pallor, cold hands and feet, depression, or, alternatively, a shortage of yang, which causes tiredness, poor circulation – all the symptoms of an underactive thyroid, in fact. Illness may also be due to a shortage of yin, which brings about insomnia, dry mouth, nervous excitement, or excess yang, characterized by heat and overactivity, a flushed face, anger, anxiety and stress – symptoms that correspond amazingly accurately to an overactive thyroid.

Visiting an Acupuncturist

An initial visit to an acupuncturist can take up to an hour. The practitioner will ask you about your health and will ask you lots of questions about aspects that might not seem immediately relevant, such as sleeping habits, preferences for different types of food, your work, lifestyle and environment.

Diagnosis is by means of the practitioner examining you for signs of the various disturbances and by taking several pulses. According to Chinese medicine, there are six pulses – three on each wrist. Each position has three depths and there are as many as 28 different pulse qualities, and checking these enables the therapist to come to a very detailed diagnosis of the condition.

The therapist will also examine your tongue, making a note of its colour, shape, thickness, moistness, and the whereabouts of any coating. He or she may also perform a physical examination.

Getting the Needle

Treatment involves inserting sterilized needles at various points along the channels in an effort to restore the body's normal balance of yin and yang and strengthen the *ch'i*. You may feel a slight pinprick as the needles are inserted or occasionally feel a tingling sensation along the channel.

Practitioners also use dried leaves of the herb mugwort, which are burned and placed around the needles to warm and tonify *ch'i* in cases where the condition is characterized by cold and damp. This technique is known as moxibustion. Alternatively a moxa stick (of burning herb) may be held close to the acupuncture point.

Reflexology

Reflexology, which involves foot and sometimes hand massage, is another therapy that relies on the concept of *ch'i* or energy.

According to reflexology teaching, there are 10 channels, beginning or ending in the toes and extending to the fingers and the top of the head. Each of these channels is associated with a particular organ of the body. The area concerned with the thyroid is at the base of the big toe, with two more points on the pads of the feet beneath and between the big toe and the next toe.

Minute crystalline deposits are said to form in areas where the energy is blocked. By massaging these points, the therapist aims to correct the energy flow and restore balance. The massage is usually gentle, but it can be momentarily uncomfortable if the practitioner presses deep into the foot. You may recall the story related earlier of the person who was prompted to seek a thyroid function test because her reflexologist detected crystals in the area linked with her thyroid.

'Glandular disease' is among the illnesses listed by one of the original proponents of reflexology, Eunice D. Ingham, in the 1930s. However, even without the potential therapeutic benefits, you may well find it tremendously relaxing and calming.

Homoeopathic Help

Homoeopathy is another therapy that may be particularly suited to thyroid problems. Like many other alternative therapies, health for a homoeopath is said to be a state of balance, and disease a result of a weakening of the body's vital force or energy. Treatment is aimed at strengthening and nourishing this vital force in order to help the body heal itself.

Remedies are based on the idea that substances which produce certain symptoms when given to a healthy person, when given to a sick one with those same symptoms, will restore health. Remedies made from plants, herbs, minerals, and other substances are repeatedly diluted and shaken or succussed – a process said to increase the power of the substance, or potentize it. As homoeopathy is aimed at a person's vital force, so the pure energy of the remedy is said to stimulate this weakened vital force. And because it is of the same nature, it is able to stimulate and nourish the vital force, which is then able to perform its job properly and restore the body to harmony.

Practitioners use what is called the law of similars to come up with various symptoms pictures, which then enable them to choose the right remedy. For example, Belladonna patients have wild, staring eyes, talk fast, are impatient, bad-tempered, irritable, and can't stand hot sun – characteristic symptoms of an overactive thyroid.

Tailored Treatment

To a homoeopath each person is different and so the same symptoms in two different people might lead to different diagnoses and treatments being given to each. For example, the symptoms of scarlet fever in one person might also point to Belladonna being prescribed, but another sufferer with scarlet fever might have a different symptom picture and, hence, need a different remedy. Thus, you can see that, because of this, diagnosis is an extremely skilled business, for all but the simplest conditions. For this reason if the idea of homeopathy appeals to you, you should visit a qualified practitioner. Some homoeopaths are also trained orthodox doctors and it may be particularly beneficial to visit such a practitioner, who will be able to monitor your progress using conventional drugs at the same time as prescribing homoeopathic remedies.

Autogenic Training

One of the few alternative therapies that has been studied specifically in relation to thyroid problems is autogenic training.

First developed in the 1920s by German doctor Wolfgang Schultz, it involves a series of exercises designed to focus the mind on feelings of heaviness, warmth in the limbs, a calm heartbeat, easy natural breathing, abdominal warmth and cooling of the forehead. You practise the exercises, sitting comfortably or lying down, three times a day, after meals, for about ten minutes.

Mild anxiety states respond particularly well to this therapy and, after four or five weeks, people are able to be gradually weaned off tranquillizers, beta-blockers, sleeping pills and other forms of medication often used to treat anxiety.

The therapy draws on some of the insights of meditation. As you focus inwardly, you leave the stresses and strains of daily life to one side for a time so that your body's own healing and relaxation abilities can be called upon to restore you.

The techniques, which are learnt initially by attending an autogenic training course, have been found to lower heart rate, blood pressure and improve emotional balance. Quite often, buried feelings of anger, grief or anxiety surface during the training. Such reactions are normal and proof that the therapy is working. The therapist can help you deal with such strong emotions and this can be enormously healing.

As far as specific thyroid symptoms are concerned, research has shown that a number of typical symptoms of an overactive thyroid, such as sweating, tremor, nausea, vomiting, diarrhoea and irritability, diminish gradually over the course of autogenic training.

Supplementary Benefits?

There's increasing interest in the use of vitamins, minerals and other nutrients to prevent and treat disease and, indeed, the links between diet and thyroid problems have been outlined elsewhere in the book. Certain substances are known as goitrogens because they interfere with iodine absorption. They most often occur in plants called brassicas, such as cabbages, turnips, and large amounts of these can cause iodine deficiency, and throw off thyroid production in those with a low-iodine intake.

There's also a link with the B vitamins. A properly functioning thyroid helps B_{12} to be absorbed. An oversupply of vitamin B_1 (thiamine) can affect thyroid and insulin production and cause loss of other B vitamins.

There's likely to be no harm in taking a daily multivitamin/mineral supplement. However, large doses of supplements should only be used cautiously, under the proper supervision of a practitioner experienced in nutritional therapy as they can affect your body in the way that drugs can and may interact with treatment for your problems. For example, vitamin E has an effect on the heart and should be used cautiously if you have an overactive thyroid, diabetes or high blood pressure.

A Word About Kelp

Kelp tablets are made from seaweed and contain iodine. In people without thyroid problems, they are said to balance the activity of the thyroid. The story is different for thyroid sufferers, however, as the amount of iodine found in various kelp preparations can't be as easily measured as it can from other sources.

By and large, iodine deficiency is no longer a problem for most of us in the West, although it's still a good idea to use sea salt in cooking and at the table. Sea fish is also a good source of iodine. Kelp, however, should be used cautiously by anyone with thyroid problems as it can provoke hyperthyroidism. It's best, therefore, not to dose yourself with kelp, and to only take it on the advice of a properly qualified herbal or nutritional practitioner.

The Feel Good Factor

As thyroid problems are so complicated, self-treatment is not recommended. Choosing an alternative therapist can be tricky though, as there are no standard qualifications as there are for orthodox practitioners. Personal recommendation can be one way to find a good therapist. Alternatively, you may want to approach one of the umbrella organizations concerned with maintaining standards in the various alternative and complementary therapies. You could also try asking your doctor to recommend someone. Increasing numbers of orthodox practitioners are now taking such therapies seriously and some even offer space to unorthodox practitioners on surgery premises. Such openness can only be a good thing.

Communication Matters

If you do decide to visit an alternative or complementary therapist, you should tell your doctor that you are doing so. A few doctors may still be resistant to the idea of complementary medicine, but, as mentioned, many doctors are beginning to recognize that unorthodox therapies can often get to the parts that conventional medicine fails to reach. Of course, if you suffer from thyroid failure, you would be unwise to place your trust exclusively in the hands of an aromatherapist, homoeopath or whatever, as only replacement of your missing hormones can restore the function of your gland. But such therapies can provide a useful adjunct to conventional treatment and help you to feel more in control of your condition, which, in turn, can help you to feel better.

Chapter 11

TOWARDS THE FUTURE

So where do we go from here? Will sufferers find it easier to be diagnosed in future, and are there any more effective treatments on the horizon?

The Great Screening Debate

Given how common thyroid problems are, an important question is whether or not doctors should be more active in trying to track down women with thyroid problems. Should doctors look for and treat 'silent' thyroid problems? And is there a case for all of us to have regular blood tests to look for signs of thyroid disease, in much the same way as we now go for a smear test?

One argument for such screening is that abnormalities in blood chemistry – evidence of silent thyroid disease – can be a clue that you will develop obvious thyroid disease in the future. Being aware of this could help you receive treatment for problems such as depression and weight gain, which are often dismissed as insignificant women's problems at the moment. It could also enable those with infertility or period problems to be picked up and treated. And it could enable women to take simple measures like strengthening the immune system by paying attention to diet or perhaps visiting a herbal practitioner, which could possibly prevent overt thyroid problems from developing. It's also argued that routine screening could save many women, like some of those whose stories we have heard in this book, from months and years of tiredness, depression and vague unwellness that are often dismissed as insignificant.

On the other hand, not everyone with silent thyroid disease goes on to develop overt thyroid disease. Is screening worth the inevitable worry that, at some vague point in the future, you might develop problems? Then again, what course should be taken in those cases where people have silent disease? Should they be actively treated or would the doctor just wait and see.

One argument *for* screening is that an underactive thyroid – even a silent one – raises cholesterol levels, which, in turn, increases the risk of developing heart disease. However, it's not yet clear whether or not permanent harm is done to the heart and blood vessels by high blood cholesterol levels in the absence of obvious hypothyroid symptoms. What's more, thyroid testing would mean even more trips to the doctor for women, who spend much more of their lives in the doctor's surgery than men do. Also, as UK endocrinologist Dr Tim Dornan writes in *GP*:

> *The screening net would have to be cast wide with repeated thyroid function testing of a large proportion of the adult population for much of adult life.*

Fifty Plus

If screening isn't introduced for *everyone*, would it be a good idea for all women over 50, say?

Thyroid problems tend to be so common as we get older anyway that they could be dubbed normal. Research suggests that thyroid cells are abnormal in most people over 60, even though they show no obvious evidence of thyroid disease. Indeed, just over one in ten elderly women have thyroid autoimmune antibodies. What's more, when examined, one in ten women in this age group have a thyroid nodule.

However, despite these figures, the decision is far from clear. On the one hand, as we've already observed, subclinical hypothyroidism could boost the risk of developing heart disease, and screening would certainly enable those at risk to be more closely monitored. Subclinical hypothyroidism is higher among women in their forties and fifties than those in their seventies and eighties, suggesting that some of the women who had it in their forties did not reach old age, perhaps as a result of their condition.

If women were screened and those with thyroid troubles were picked up, should those at risk be given thyroxine? Some doctors think so. On the other hand, as US doctors Mark Helfand and Lawrence M. Crapo point out in an article in the *Annals of Internal Medicine* (June 1990), no one knows what the long-term risks of taking thyroxine are in cases of silent disease. It's possible that it could actually aggravate existing heart problems and, as we've seen, it can thin the bones, leading to an increased risk of osteoporosis. What's more, it would mean that many perfectly well women would be taking possibly unnecessary drugs. They add, 'Presently the balance between the short-term benefits and potential long-term risks cannot be estimated.'

So, the jury is still out. However, some doctors, such as UK endocrinologist Dr Tim Dornan, favour what they describe as 'opportunistic testing', which is, for example, testing women with vague symptoms, such as depression and weight gain, and routine testing of those with infertility problems, menstrual irregularities and elderly women who are obviously unwell. And screening could be worthwhile in the future if new preventative treatments are developed – something that could well be on the cards.

Finding the Cause

As experts get ever closer to tracking down the root causes of thyroid disease, we can certainly expect to see improved ways of treatment. As we have seen elsewhere, investigations into the immune connection are yielding some particularly fascinating insights. It's becoming increasingly clear that much thyroid disease – particularly where Graves' and Hashimoto's are found in the same family – has genetic origins. New research into the interplay between genes and the environment could lead to some promising new treatments. Professor Weetman, a UK expert, says, 'We're not going to find a single gene: it's more like a fruit machine – you'll get several lemons, both genetic and environmental'.

As long ago as 1982, researchers suggested that autoimmune disease in older sufferers was more likely to be laid at the door of environmental factors, while in children a similar disease is more likely to be attributable to inherited genes.

To test this, researchers analysed the families of a group of children and teenagers suffering from Hashimoto's disease to see whether or not the genetic predisposition was mirrored by a high number of autoantibodies in close relatives, such as brothers, sisters and parents. Sure enough, they found that, in Hashimoto's sufferers, close relatives were more likely themselves to possess thyroid autoantibodies than average. As a result of this research and a growing body of other studies, scientists have come to believe that thyroid antibodies are a dominant trait (one that is inherited if either one of the parents possesses it) that confers a susceptibility to developing thyroid disease, especially in women.

Using more sensitive tests, other researchers have found strong evidence that genes involved in regulating T cells (white blood cells that patrol the body and repel any invaders) are important factors in dictating the development of disease in those who are susceptible.

Yet another piece of the jigsaw could be added by another research study, which showed that there is a particularly high prevalence of thyroid autoimmunity in relatives of families with Alzheimer's disease and Down's syndrome. Down's syndrome is caused by there being three copies, instead of the normal pair, of chromosome 21. Professor Weetman observes:

> *Both Alzheimer's and Down's are due to aberrations on chromosome 21. The implication is that this chromosome has an influence on the development of thyroid disease. It could be a direct influence, in that the same chromosome could be responsible for thyroid disease, or it could be indirect in that the chromosome controls the immune system in general.*

Are Infections to Blame?

As we've seen throughout this book, genes may load the gun of autoimmunity, but factors in the environment are required to pull the trigger. One such triggering factor may be infection. Many aspects of modern life, such as poor digestion and absorption, poor diet, toxins, the side-effects of medicines and stress can all lower immune resistance and make us prone to minor infections. As we've seen, the food poisoning bug yersinia has been found to be involved in Graves' disease. Hepatitis C is another potential culprit. It causes a mild flu-like illness and, though it can be caught from the blood of an infected carrier, through sharing toothbrushes, razors or needles, in four out of ten cases the cause is unknown.

Another piece of research, reported by Professor Weetman in *Clinical Endocrinology* in 1992, found that the Epstein-Barr virus was implicated in the development of autoimmune thyroiditis in three patients. Intriguingly, this is the same virus that causes glandular fever and has been implicated in ME, otherwise known as chronic fatigue. So, could there be a connection between chronic fatigue and hypothyroidism? Clearly, three patients isn't enough of a sample from which to draw any firm conclusions, but it is an intriguing suggestion and could lead researchers yet another step nearer to finding the underlying cause.

The suggestion that infection may be involved is supported by some other research, also reported by Professor Weetman, on strains of rats prone to develop thyroiditis. But, in this case, the source was micro-organisms that normally live in the gut without causing problems. Some experiments designed to encourage the development of thyroiditis in the rats were set up. These experiments showed that animals raised in a germ-free environment didn't develop the disease, whereas those infected with germs from the guts of other (normal) rats did.

Weetman comments that, although we should be cautious in drawing hard and fast conclusions from the research, this could point to a possible role for germs that normally dwell in the body without causing any problems as opposed to infectious agents from outside.

Unfortunately, attractive though the suggestion is, there's still no hard evidence that infections are definitely involved in autoimmune thyroid problems, but it's certainly an area that warrants further research. If it does turn out to be the case, building up our immune systems so that we are more resistant could well help.

Environmental Poisons

Another question mark lies over the question of whether or not environmental toxins, such as pesticides, food additives and pollution, could play a part in the development of autoimmunity. Doctors known as clinical ecologists, who are concerned with the effects of the environment on disease, have long claimed that such factors are to blame in a vast number of illnesses, while conventional doctors have tended to dismiss such links. However, in one piece of research carried out in 1991, Professor Weetman found that certain products derived from coal tar (anthracene), sparked off autoimmune thyroid problems in certain genetically susceptible strains of rats. Coal tar derivatives are used in some dyes and food additives, so could the environmentalists be right after all? No one knows, but Weetman comments:

> *It seems likely that a combination of genetic, constitutional and environmental factors initiate autoimmune thyroiditis [though] the relative contribution of each of these, and almost certainly of undiscovered factors, is unknown.*

Future Positive?

So, what of the future? And what do the various debates and new research mean to thyroid sufferers? The experts clearly have much more to learn about thyroid problems. Professor Weetman concludes that, in the main, the research described won't make that much difference to most thyroid sufferers. He says:

> *In terms of hypothyroid problems I can't see any improvement on thyroxine. It's safe and cheap. I know it's a chore to take tablets every day, but it's natural, it doesn't have side effects – I can't conceive of an easier way.*

This said, all the research that is going on could greatly improve the quality of life for sufferers from autoimmune thyroid disease, one of the most important causes of thyroid problems, and, in particular, those with thyroid eye disease, which is still an enigma.

On the genetic front, gene hunters are now trying to track down potentially faulty genes in groups of families using 'probes' to search for specific markers in the blood, which might indicate the whereabouts of potential culprits. Other researchers are on the track of finding environmental triggers, such as diet, infection, pollution and so on, that might damage the cells and lead to the development of thyroid problems. Such research will almost certainly lead to more sophisticated treatments that are designed to stem the disease process itself, especially for those with an overactive thyroid, rather than the somewhat crude treatments used at present.

It could certainly be argued that it would be better to treat, or even better prevent, the underlying disease process rather than relying on the hit-and-miss method of reducing the manufacture and secretion of thyroid hormones, radioactive iodine or surgery.

Such treatments might include developing monoclonal antibodies, artificial antibodies that are designed to hone in on particular foreign cells. Other treatments could involve the development of antagonists – drugs that work by preventing antigens from binding to receptors and so block the cell's response.

One possibility is that, at some time in the future, such treatments could be developed into a vaccine to prevent thyroid problems in those at risk. Professor Weetman explains:

> *If you take the T cells that cause disease and treat them in such a way that it prevents them causing disease for example by irradiating them and then reintroduce them into the body, that 'vaccine' will prevent the disease occurring. Alternatively receptors that recognize the T cells could be produced as a 'vaccine'. Even more subtly if you take bits of protein from the thyroid, you can trick the immune cells into not responding.*

However any such vaccine would need to be given right at the beginning of the disease, something that could be difficult to pinpoint given the insidious way in which thyroid disease tends to creep up on people.

The only way this could be achieved would be to have some

sort of screening programme, perhaps testing those at risk because of a family history of thyroid problems, to check for the first hint of disease. However, given the big debate on whether or not thyroid disease should be screened for, this raises many questions. Professor Weetman observes, 'It might be possible to do this for Grave's disease. It's been looked at mainly for diabetes and MS, but I suspect it won't be done for thyroid disease.'

Such treatments are still, of course, some way in the future, but the fact that thyroid disease is at last being taken more seriously should mean some potentially more effective treatments on the horizon. In the meantime, if you've got this far, you will realize that thyroid disease doesn't have to rule your life – there are plenty of ways in which you can help yourself when you have thyroid disease. Experimenting with these should enable you to feel a renewed sense of energy and vigour so that you can live a healthy, active life, despite your illness.

Appendix

Where to Find Out More

Useful Addresses

Thyroid Problems
British Thyroid Foundation
PO Box HP22
Leeds LS6 3RT

Thyroid Eye Disease
Lea House
21 Troarn Way
Chudleigh
Devon TQ13 0PP

MedicAlert
12 Bridge Wharf
156 Caledonian Road
London N1 9UU

Weight Problems and/or Eating Disorders
Eating Disorders Association
Sackville Place
44 Magdalen Street
Norwich NR3 1JU

Emotional Problems

Women's Therapy Centre
6–9 Manor Gardens
London N7 6LA

Alternative Therapies

British Complementary Medicine Association
St Charles Hospital
Exmoor Street
London W10 6DZ

Institute for Complementary Medicine
60 Great Ormond Street
London WC1N 3RH

Further Reading

Bayliss, Dr R., and Tunbridge, Dr W. M., *Thyroid Disease: The Facts*, Oxford University Press, 1991

Fulder, Dr Stephen, *How to Survive Medical Treatment*, The C. W. Daniel Company Limited, 1994

Gomez, Dr Joan, *Coping with Thyroid Problems*, Sheldon Press, 1994

Hillson, Dr Rowan, *Thyroid Disorders*, Optima, 1991

Kirsta, Alex, *The Book of Stress Survival*, Gaia Books, 1986

Nagarathna, Dr R., Nagendra, Dr H. R., and Monro, Dr Robin, *Yoga for Common Ailments*, Gaia Books, 1990

van Straten, Michael, and Griggs, Barbara, *Superfoods*, Dorling Kindersley, 1992

INDEX